WORLD HEALTH ORGANIZATION

C000115177

The

WORLD
HEALTH
REPORT
1999

Making a Difference

WHO Library Cataloguing in Publication Data

The world health report 1999: Making a difference
1. World health – trends   2. Health priorities   3. Cost of illness
4. Health services accessibility   5. Social justice   6. Poverty
7. Forecasting   8. Mortality – trends   9. Malaria – prevention and control
10. Smoking – prevention and control   11. World Health Organization
I. Title: Making a difference

ISBN 92 4 156194 7   (NLM Classification: WA 540.1)
ISSN 1020-3311

The World Health Organization welcomes requests for permission to reproduce or translate its publications, in part or in full. Applications and enquiries should be addressed to the Office of Publications, World Health Organization, 1211 Geneva 27, Switzerland, which will be glad to provide the latest information on any changes made to the text, plans for new editions, and reprints and translations already available.

© **World Health Organization 1999**
All rights reserved.

The designations employed and the presentation of the material in this publication, including tables and maps, do not imply the expression of any opinion whatsoever on the part of the Secretariat of the World Health Organization concerning the legal status of any country, territory, city or area or of its authorities, or concerning the delimitation of its frontiers or boundaries. Dotted lines on maps represent approximate border lines for which there may not yet be full agreement.

The mention of specific companies or of certain manufacturers' products does not imply that they are endorsed or recommended by the World Health Organization in preference to others of a similar nature that are not mentioned. Errors and omissions excepted, the names of proprietary products are distinguished by initial capital letters.

Information concerning this publication can be obtained from:
World Health Report
World Health Organization
1211 Geneva 27, Switzerland
Fax: (41-22) 791 4870

This report was prepared by Dean T. Jamison, Andrew Creese and Thomson Prentice, with the assistance of a core team composed of Emmanuela Gakidou, Mie Inoue, and Michel Beusenberg. Other contributors were, in alphabetical order, Howard Engers, Catherine Goodman, Emmanuel Guidon, Prabhat Jha, Kamini Mendis, David Nabarro, Jim Tulloch, Jia Wang, and Derek Yach. Comments were appreciated from a number of individuals including Anarfi Asamoah-Baah, David Evans, Tore Godal, Joseph Kutzin, Alan Lopez, Christopher Murray, Richard Peto and Nicholas White; additional help was gratefully received from WHO Regional Directors, Executive Directors and their respective staffs.

Administrative support was provided by Aquilina John-Mutaboyerwa and Shelagh Probst. The report was edited by Barbara Campanini and Angela Haden, and translated into French by Barbara Audrin and Jean-Claude Guyonnet. The index was prepared by Liza Weinkove and, for the French edition, by Laurent Gaiddon.

The report was prepared under the general direction of Jonas Støre, Executive Director, Director-General's Office, and Senior Policy Adviser; Julio Frenk, Executive Director, Evidence and Information for Policy; and Susan Holck, Director of Health Information Management and Dissemination.

The cover painting "Working Woman", by Mr Nuwa Wamala-Nnyanzi, of the Nnyanzi Studio and Gallery of African Art, Kampala, Uganda, is reproduced with the kind permission of the artist.

Design by Marilyn Langfeld. Layout by WHO Graphics
Printed in France
99/12368 – Sadag – 20000

CONTENTS

INDEX   117

TABLES

FIGURES

Boxes

MESSAGE FROM
THE DIRECTOR-GENERAL

*I*n May of this year, health ministers and leaders from around the world will gather in Geneva for the final World Health Assembly of the century. This year's *World health report – Making a difference* reviews the accomplishments and challenges in world health and highlights their implications for WHO's approach, priorities and work in the years to come.

The world enters the 21st century with hope but also with uncertainty. Remarkable gains in health, rapid economic growth and unprecedented scientific advance – all legacies of the 20th century – could lead us to a new era of human progress. But darker legacies bring uncertainty to this vision – and demand redoubled commitment. Regional conflicts have replaced the global wars of the first half of the 20th century as a source of continued misery. Deep poverty remains all too prevalent. The sustainability of a healthy environment is still unproved. The Universal Declaration of Human Rights – now half a century old – is only a tantalizing promise for far too many of our fellow humans. The HIV/AIDS epidemic continues unchecked in much of the world, and it warns us against complacency about other, still unknown, microbial threats.

We can make a difference. Those of us who commit our lives to improving health can help to make sure

Dr Gro Harlem Brundtland

that hope will predominate over uncertainty in the century to come. Human health – and its influence on every aspect of life – is central to the larger picture.

With vision, commitment and successful leadership, this report argues, the world could end the first decade of the 21st century with notable accomplishments. Many of the world's poor people would no longer suffer today's burden of premature death and excessive disability, and poverty itself would thereby be much reduced. Healthy life expectancy would increase for all. Smoking and other risks to health would fade in significance. The financial burdens of medical needs would be more fairly shared, leaving no household without access to care or exposed to economic ruin as a result of health expenditure. And health systems would respond with greater compassion, quality and efficiency to the increasingly diverse demands they face. Progress in the 20th century points to the real opportunity for reaching these goals.

Opportunity entails responsibility. Working together we have the opportunity to transform lives now debilitated by disease and fear of economic ruin into lives filled with realistic hopes. I have pledged to place health at the core of the global development agenda. That is where it belongs. Wise investments in health can prove to be the most successful strategies to lead people out of poverty.

This report argues that improvements in health have contributed to spur human and economic development in the past – and that this will also prove true in the future.

I have always believed that you cannot make real changes in society unless the economic dimension of the issue is fully understood. I firmly believe that this is what took "the environment" from being a cause for the committed few to becoming a societal issue for the attention of major players. The scientific facts were gathered. The true costs of environmental degradation were analysed and enumerated in figures. Then, gradually, governments and parliaments started to vote incentives to change behavioural patterns among industry and consumers. There is still far to go in the field of environment and sustainable development, but the trend has been started.

A new trend may be set in motion as we see and understand the broader implications of poverty. For the World Health Organization this means real inspiration. We intend to collect, analyse and spread the evidence that investing in health is one major avenue towards poverty alleviation.

We must be realistic: there will be setbacks and difficulties. A greater collective effort will generate more demands on each of us individually and on the institutions we represent – national and international, public and private. Compressing the time required to accomplish major and tangible results is the task for leadership in the 21st century. This leadership must be technical. It must be political. And it must be moral.

PROGRESS AND CHALLENGES

An historic conference in Alma-Ata in 1978 established the goal of Health for All by the year 2000. It defined this goal as "the attainment by all peoples of the world by the year 2000 of a level of health that will permit them to lead a socially and economically productive life". This report describes how the past few decades – the period following the Declaration of Alma-Ata – have witnessed revolutionary gains in life expectancy. These gains build on progress that began for some countries in the late 19th century. Among today's high income countries, life expectancy increased by 30 to 40 years in this century. Most of today's low and middle income countries have experienced even more dramatic gains, although remaining inequalities needlessly burden disadvantaged populations and prolong their poverty. Under WHO's leadership the world eradicated smallpox, one of the most devastating diseases of history, and today a substantial majority of the world's population faces relatively low risk from infectious diseases of any sort.

These health gains have transformed quality of life and created conditions favouring sustained fertility reductions and consequent demographic change. In many developing countries, for example, the total fertility rate – the expected number of children a woman will bear over her lifetime – declined from over six in the late 1950s to about three at present. These health and demographic changes have contributed directly to the global diffusion of rapid economic growth that, like the health revolution, constitutes an extraordinary accomplishment of the century now closing.

In an important sense, then, the world has made great progress towards better Health for All. Inspiration and guidance from Alma-Ata, with its major emphasis on the critical role of primary health care, contributed in no small measure to the health revolution. Continued improvement in living standards has also played a role. More important, though, has probably been the generation and application of new knowledge about diseases and their control. These factors have yielded substantial success by any measure, but problems and challenges remain.

Some problems emerge from the reduction in mortality from infectious disease and accompanying declines in fertility: the very successes of the past few decades will, inexorably, generate a "demographic transition" from traditional societies where almost everyone is young to societies with rapidly increasing numbers of the middle-aged and elderly. With this transition a new set of diseases rises to prominence: cancers, heart disease, stroke and mental illness figure prominently among them. Available interventions against these diseases, including preventive ones, yield less decisive results than we have achieved for most infectious diseases. And their costs can be very high indeed.

Furthermore, as this report documents, over a billion people will enter the 21st century without having benefited from the health revolution: their lives remain short and scarred by disease. Many countries must deal with these disease problems of the poor while simultaneously responding to rapid growth in noncommunicable diseases: they face a double burden. Large numbers of other individuals, while not poor, fail to realize their full potential for better health because health systems allocate resources to interventions of low quality or of low efficacy related to cost. Increasing numbers of people forego or defer essential care or suffer huge financial burdens resulting from an unexpected need for expensive services. The continuing challenges to health ministries and to countries thus remain enormous. New problems constantly arise: witness the emergence of the HIV epidemic, the threat of resurgent malaria or the unexpected magnitude and consequences of the tobacco epidemic. Achieving better health for all is an ever-changing task. Success will make a major difference in the quality of life worldwide. And the difference for the poor will be not only in improving their quality of life but also, through increasing their productivity, in addressing one of the root causes of poverty.

Global leadership and advocacy for health remain critical missing ingredients in the formula for making a difference and conveying evidence to the highest level of government. We need to remind prime ministers and finance ministers that they are health ministers themselves and that investments in the health of the poor can enhance growth and reduce poverty. Leadership must motivate and guide the technical community to bring today's powerful tools to bear on the challenges before us.

Let us review the challenges to be addressed in order to improve the world's health.

- First and foremost, *there is a need to reduce greatly the burden of excess mortality and morbidity suffered by the poor.* The OECD's Development Assistance Committee has established the target of halving the number of people living in absolute poverty by the year 2015. This goal is attainable, but it will require major shifts in the way that governments all over the world use their resources. It will mean focusing more on interventions that we know can achieve the greatest health gain possible within prevailing resource limits. It will mean giving renewed attention to diseases like tuberculosis, which disproportionately affect poor people, as well as malaria and HIV/AIDS, which we now recognize as major constraints to economic growth.

  Women and children suffer poverty more than men: there is therefore a need for greater investment in reducing maternal mortality – and finding ways of improving maternal and childhood nutrition. Reducing the burden of excess mortality and morbidity also means revitalizing and extending the coverage of immunization programmes – still one of the most powerful and cost-effective technologies at our disposal. The elimination of poliomyelitis in the Americas in the past decade, and great progress in control elsewhere, hold out the promise that polio will join smallpox as a disease known only to history.

The new focus on reducing the burden of disease suffered by poor people is not just a call to governments alone. To make real inroads into absolute poverty will mean harnessing the energies and resources of the private sector and civil society as well. We need to be clear about what the world should be aiming to achieve and the resources needed to achieve global goals. We believe there is a good case for negotiating realistic national and international targets as a means of mobilizing resources, concentrating international attention on the most important problems, and ensuring proper monitoring of progress and achievement.

- Second, *there is a need to counter potential threats to health* resulting from economic crises, unhealthy environments or risky behaviour. Tobacco addiction is one of the single most important threats. It is not just an issue for the north: over 80% of all smokers today live in developing countries. A global commitment to tobacco control can potentially avert scores of millions of premature deaths in the next half century, and its success can point the way for effective control of other threats.

  Preparing effective responses to emerging infections and countering the spread of resistance to antimicrobials will help insure against the prospect of a significantly increased infectious disease threat. Beyond countering specific threats, promotion of healthy lifestyles underpins a proactive strategy for risk reduction: cleaner air and water, adequate sanitation, healthy diets and safer transportation – all are important. And all are facilitated by stable economic growth and by ensuring that females as well as males have opportunities to increase their educational attainment.

- Third, *there is a need to develop more effective health systems.* In many parts of the world, health systems are ill-equipped to cope with present demands, let alone those they will face in the future. The institutional problems which limit health sector performance are often common to all public services in a country. But, despite their importance, they have been relatively neglected by governments and development agencies alike.

  We now recognize that dealing with issues such as pay and incentives in the public sector, priority setting and rationing, and unregulated growth in the private sector constitute some of the most challenging items on the international health agenda.

  The report's chapter on health systems development points to change taking place in all parts of the world – change that responds to different problems in different ways. The pressure for change provides the opportunity for reform. But reform requires a sense of direction. In my view, the broad goal of better health for all should guide reform. Beyond this, however, there is a need to be clear about the desirable characteristics of health systems. The goal must be to create health systems that can:
  - improve health status;
  - reduce health inequalities;
  - enhance responsiveness to legitimate expectations;
  - increase efficiency;
  - protect individuals, families and communities from financial loss;
  - enhance fairness in the financing and delivery of health care.

Limits exist on what governments can finance and on their capacity to deliver services and to regulate the private sector. Hence the need for public policies that recognize these limits. Governments should retain responsibility for setting broad policy directions, for creating an appropriate regulatory environment, and for finance. At the same time they should seek both to diversify the sources of service provision and to select interventions that, for the resources each country chooses to commit, will provide the maximum gains in health levels and their most equitable distribution. At an international level we need, collectively, to improve our capacity for humanitarian assistance and for responding to complex emergencies, when national health systems cannot cope.

- Finally, *there is a need to invest in expanding the knowledge base* that made the 20th century revolution in health possible, and that will provide the tools for continued gains in the 21st century. Governments of high income countries and large, research-oriented pharmaceutical companies now invest – and will continue to invest – massive resources in research and development oriented to the needs of the more affluent.

  Much of this investment benefits all humanity, but at least two critical gaps remain. One concerns research and development relevant to the infectious diseases that overwhelmingly afflict the poor. The other concerns the systematic generation of an information base that countries can use in shaping the future of their own health systems.

A CORPORATE STRATEGY FOR WHO

The challenges outlined above constitute an agenda for the world community as a whole: for governments and development agencies alike. Even as the lead agency in health, we have to recognize that the agenda is too broad for WHO alone. We therefore have to be realistic, and start to define how WHO can contribute most effectively to this agenda in coming years.

We intend that four interconnected strategic themes should guide the work of the whole Organization. The first two concern *where* we focus our efforts. The second two concern *how* we work. These are the themes that must guide our work:
- we need to be more focused in improving health outcomes;
- we need to be more effective in supporting health systems development;
- we need to be more impact-oriented in our work with countries;
- we need to be more innovative in creating influential partnerships.

IMPROVING HEALTH OUTCOMES

This theme runs through everything we do. Our first priority must be to reduce – then eliminate – the debilitating excess burden of disease among the poor. I am particularly concerned that we focus on health interventions that will help lead populations out of poverty. Let me highlight some key priorities as they are defined in the *Proposed Budget 2000-2001.*
- We are committed to reducing the burden of sickness and suffering resulting from communicable diseases. Roll Back Malaria is central to this approach. But we will also contribute as effectively as possible to combating the global epidemics of HIV/AIDS and tuberculosis, and to completing the eradication of poliomyelitis.
- We need to step up our ability to deal with the rising toll of noncommunicable diseases. Special attention will be given to cancer and cardiovascular diseases. The Tobacco Free

Initiative is supporting and leading this approach.
- We will pay more attention to the delivery of high quality health care for children, adolescents and women.
- WHO is committed to making progress on the issues of population and reproductive health – with a special focus on maternal mortality and adolescent sexual and reproductive health.
- We will put the spotlight back on immunization as one of the most cost-effective health interventions.
- We need to intensify our efforts to reduce the enormous burden of malnutrition, especially in children.
- We will continue to support countries in their quest for access to affordable and high quality essential drugs.
- We will work to see that mental health – and particularly the neglected scourge of depression – is given the attention it deserves.
- We need to be better at responding to increasingly diverse kinds of emergencies and humanitarian crises.
- We will develop our capacity within WHO – and in collaboration with others – to give advice on crucial health care financing issues.
- And we need to be able to deal more effectively with intersectoral issues – particularly the threats to health that result from environmental causes.

Let me focus on two of our key initiatives: Roll Back Malaria and the Tobacco Free Initiative. *The world health report 1999* devotes a chapter to each of these.

Malaria and underdevelopment are closely intertwined. Over 40% of the world's population live where there is a risk of malaria. The disease causes widespread premature death and suffering, imposes financial hardship on poor households, and holds back economic growth and improvements in living standards. Malaria flourishes in situations of social and environmental crisis, weak health systems and disadvantaged communities.

Its ability to develop resistance makes malaria a formidable adversary. Available and effective interventions – such as insecticide-treated bednets – fail to reach the people with the greatest burden of malaria. Capacity for malaria control is inadequate in endemic countries, where health systems are often weak. Better implementation of current knowledge, and new products and technologies are all needed to break down the barrier to human progress which malaria poses. Overcoming these problems is a challenge for leadership, a challenge to be met by the Roll Back Malaria project.

Successful malaria control involves strengthening health systems. Weak health systems and uninvolved communities are part of the malaria problem. Because malaria is an acute condition with a rapid natural history, easy access to health care of good quality is vital in its management. Externally driven initiatives, by-passing local and national health systems, are neither sustainable nor supportive of malaria control and health development. Many countries have begun the process of reforming their health system to improve performance. Malaria control, like the better management of all illnesses, needs to build on and support these changes. Through strengthened health systems, total malaria deaths could be halved – 500 000 deaths could be averted annually – for about U$1 billion per year of additional spending.

A new willingness to collaborate has been demonstrated. The Organization of African Unity, the World Bank and WHO's African Region have already planned a major African Initiative on Malaria which is expected to spearhead Roll Back Malaria in Africa. Roll Back

Malaria differs from previous efforts to fight malaria. It will work to create new tools for controlling malaria, and by strengthening health systems for sustainable health improvement. Roll Back Malaria will also act as a pathfinder, helping to set the direction and strategy for more integrated action in other priority areas, such as tuberculosis control and safe motherhood. Greater reliance on partnerships in fighting malaria will inform WHO's approach to other major health challenges and to the development of effective coordinated multipartner action.

Momentum for action against malaria has been increasing fast. Strong political support has come from the Organization of African Unity and the G8 group of the most industrialized countries. Four international agencies with major concerns about malaria and its effects on health and the economy – UNICEF, the United Nations Development Programme, the World Bank and the World Health Organization – agreed, at a meeting of agency heads in October 1998, jointly to support Roll Back Malaria with WHO leadership.

Let me now turn to the Tobacco Free Initiative. The tobacco epidemic claims a large and rapidly growing number of premature deaths every year. Our estimates suggest that in 1998 the world suffered about 4 million tobacco-related deaths; to put this slightly differently, about one in twelve adult deaths in 1990 resulted from tobacco use and, by 2020, tobacco will cause as many as one in seven. Perhaps 70% of these will be in the developing world. Millions more suffer from disabling lung or heart disease, impotence or impaired pregnancies.

This tobacco toll is now growing most rapidly in developing countries. Can the momentum of the epidemic be slowed? Have government policies been able to counter the marketing strength of the industry and the addictive powers of nicotine? The record here is clear: effective control strategies exist and governments that have adopted them have succeeded in reducing tobacco use. The challenge is to transform ongoing successes into far more comprehensive global efforts.

At the same time that it is saving lives, tobacco control will also save money. Resources committed to tobacco production will be freed, but as this is at best a gradual process today's producers will suffer few transition costs. Consumer "benefits" from tobacco use accrue substantially to addiction – addiction acquired for most smokers while they were children or young teenagers. A recent and comprehensive World Bank review concludes unequivocally that tobacco control results in net economic as well as health benefits.

What lessons have we learned concerning the design of effective anti-tobacco strategies? This report concludes that effective action rests on four principles of control:

- providing public health information through media and schools, and banning tobacco advertising and promotion;
- using taxes and regulations to reduce consumption;
- encouraging cessation of tobacco use in part by encouraging less harmful and less expensive ways of delivering controlled and diminishing quantities of nicotine;
- building anti-tobacco coalitions and defusing opposition to control measures.

These measures cost relatively little and, through tobacco taxes, can more than finance themselves. Each contributes to the control agenda, and typically each would be included in national control strategies.

Yet how best to design the implementation of these measures in a national or local context is still a puzzle; how to counter the opposition of the multinational tobacco industry remains a constant challenge; and how to tap the global moral, intellectual and political commitment to tobacco control for advancing a national agenda is often an unanswered question. No central point has existed for accumulating the experience of what does and does not work – or for mobilizing political, legal and financial resources to assist governments or elements of civil society that are committed to tobacco control. It was to fill these gaps – to provide the requisite leadership – that we launched the global Tobacco Free Initiative on 21 July 1998. A major milestone for the initiative will be the adoption of a "Framework Convention on Tobacco Control" by 2003, and initial efforts towards this are well under way.

SUPPORTING HEALTH SECTOR DEVELOPMENT

WHO has always been strong at responding to specific requests. The Organization is good at fielding highly qualified technical experts. But often individual experts tend to see the world through their own expert lenses. WHO has, however, been less good at helping senior decision-makers deal with the big picture.

We know that senior policy-makers in ministries of health do not have the luxury of focusing on single issues. Health is one of the most politically and institutionally difficult sectors in any country. If WHO is to earn a leadership role in health, we cannot deny the responsibility of helping our colleagues to deal with complexity.

In many countries, national governments have tended to look to other agencies for advice on issues that affect the sector as a whole. WHO has to be a more reliable and effective supporter of countries as they reform and restructure their health sectors. We also have to be clear that reform is not an end in itself. It is a way of making sure that people – particularly poor people – get a better deal from their health system.

Many determinants of better health lie outside the health system altogether: they lie in better education (and in ensuring that girls have the same educational opportunities as boys). They lie in cleaner environments, and in sustained reductions in poverty. We must understand these linkages. One path to better health for all is for those of us within the health sector to serve as active and informed advocates of health-friendly policies outside the sector.

The second path is through reform of health systems themselves. Reform today, in much of the world, will take place in a context of increased reliance on the market forces which have increased productivity in many sectors of the world economy. But markets have failed to achieve similar success in health services or health insurance. At the same time, many of the new products critical to improving health originate in the private sector. Active government involvement in providing universal health care has contributed to the great gains of recent years – but many governments have overextended themselves. Efforts to provide all services to all people have led to arbitrary rationing, inequities, nonresponsiveness and inadequate finance for essential services.

Where, then, do the values of WHO lead when combined with the available evidence? *They cannot lead to a form of public intervention that has governments attempting to provide and finance everything for everybody.* This "classical" universalism, although seldom advanced in extreme form, shaped the formation of many well-established health systems. It achieved important successes. But the old universalism fails to recognize both resource limits and the limits of government.

Our values cannot support market-oriented approaches that ration health services to those with the ability to pay. Not only do market-oriented approaches lead to intolerable inequity with respect to a fundamental human right, but growing bodies of theory and evidence indicate markets in health to be inefficient as well. Market mechanisms have enormous utility in many sectors and have underpinned rapid economic growth for over a century in

Europe and elsewhere. But the very countries that have relied heavily on market mechanisms to achieve the high incomes they enjoy today are the same countries that rely most heavily on governments to finance health services.

With the exception of only the United States, the high income market-oriented democracies mandate universal coverage. Their health outcomes are very high. They have contained expenditures to a much smaller fraction of GDP than has the USA (7–10% versus 14%). In the one country where it was studied – Canada – introduction of National Health Insurance resulted in increased wages, reduced unemployment and improved health outcomes. Therein lies a lesson.

This report advocates a "new universalism" that recognizes governments' limits but retains government responsibility for leadership, regulation and finance of health systems. The new universalism welcomes diversity and, subject to appropriate guidelines, competition in the provision of services. At the same time it recognizes that if services are to be provided for all then not all services can be provided. The most cost-effective services should be provided first. The new universalism welcomes private sector involvement in supplying service providers with drugs and equipment, and encourages increased public and private investment in generating the new drugs, equipment and vaccines that will underpin long-term improvements in health. But it entrusts the public sector with the fundamental responsibility of ensuring solidarity in financing health care for all. It further calls for a strategic reorientation of ministries of health towards stewardship of the entire system through participatory, fair and efficient regulation.

Countries approach WHO with concerns about health finance broadly defined, more than on any other question. Our thinking in this area generally reflects this new universalism. We are rapidly building internal capacity to learn about health finance and to respond more effectively to questions concerning it.

Regaining our place at the centre of the health sector development agenda is a challenge for the whole of WHO; it is one reason why I have launched a project under the title of Partnerships for Health Sector Development. The project will be working to advance our strategic agenda on several fronts. It will work throughout the Organization to establish a health sector development perspective in all aspects of our work. It will also be concerned to help to develop a more strategic approach to work with countries. In addition, the project will have a role in establishing more influential partnerships.

A MORE STRATEGIC APPROACH TO OUR WORK IN AND WITH COUNTRIES

The financial resources for health lie overwhelmingly *within* countries. Responsibility for success (or failure) thus lies ultimately with governments. Only a tiny fraction of resources for health in low and middle income countries originates in the international system – development banks, bilateral development assistance agencies, international nongovernmental organizations, foundations and WHO. Health spending in low and middle income countries in 1994 totalled about $250 billion, of which only $2 or 3 billion was from development assistance. We also need to recognize that WHO is not a donor agency. Its prime resources are knowledge and people. In thinking about our relationships with Member States, we need to think not just about what we spend but about what we *do*.

We work for countries in two ways. We work *in* countries by establishing a direct presence to respond to national developmental needs. In this regard, it is essential that our in-country presence is adequate for the tasks we need to undertake. We also work *with* the entire community of countries, collectively or in groups, helping them to mobilize their collective wisdom, knowledge and efforts in the production of norms and standards, sound evidence and surveillance data. These are all international public goods which benefit all.

In allocating our resources to country-specific work, concentrating technical assistance on countries with a shared strategic vision will enhance impact. We have a clear mandate adopted by our Member States – and the World Health Assembly regularly votes recommendations and policies which we are pursuing – so we should support related projects and policies to which governments are committed, rather than attempting to impose an outsider's perspective.

Concentrating resources on poor countries or vulnerable groups without alternative sources of finance will also amplify our impact. A recent World Bank review of what works in development assistance – and of what fails – found strong support for these conclusions. When development assistance was used to support governments with sound policies it contributed significantly to economic growth and poverty reduction, particularly in poorer countries. But when external actors pushed against the grain of weak national policies they failed. The review further concluded that far too much development assistance has indeed been wasted for just this reason.

If WHO is to make a difference the implication is clear: concentrate country-specific technical assistance for health on countries whose policies reflect a shared vision of reaching the poor and of efficiency in health systems development. But as a technical agency committed to improve the health of the poor, we also need to focus on vulnerable populations and do what we can to help to improve their health status.

The second modality for focusing our country efforts involves working with the entire community of countries. The international community should avoid using its resources for what individual countries can do for themselves. International resources should, instead, concentrate on functions that require international collective action. These tasks include:
- global leadership and advocacy for health;
- generating and disseminating an evidence and information base for all countries to use;
- catalyzing effective global disease surveillance (as is currently done with influenza, to take one important example);
- setting norms and standards;
- targeting specific global or regional health problems where the concerted action of countries is required (for example, eradication of poliomyelitis);
- helping to provide a voice for those whose health is neglected within their own country or who are stateless;
- ensuring that critical research and development for the poor receives finance.

Each of these tasks involves working with the community of nations.

I wish to see a shift in the way WHO thinks and acts in its work with countries. Let us reflect for a moment on what it will take for our Organization to enhance its contribution.
- WHO needs to be seen by governments and other agencies to have a sound understanding of sectoral needs and the political and institutional contexts in which they have to be addressed.
- WHO needs to be a reliable source of high quality advice, and to act as a facilitator with

a technically authoritative voice.

- WHO needs to possess up-to-date and relevant evidence, set relevant norms and standards, and be responsive to the needs of Member States.
- WHO should be able to serve as a broker and negotiator for better health – helping to reconcile concerns and needs of Member States and external agencies that support the health sector.
- WHO should be able to help to shape the rules of engagement between governments and external agencies, as well as being able to use its own limited financial resources as strategically as possible.
- WHO should be instrumental not only in raising international resources for health, but also in placing health at the heart of the development agenda.

This is a tall order. But it is a clear and consistent message, one that comes from all our international partners, and is a sound reminder for the renewal process.

FORGING MORE INFLUENTIAL PARTNERSHIPS

In approaching partnerships, we need to shift our strategic direction substantially. We need to move from our traditional approach – which too often has favoured our own small-scale projects – to one which gives more emphasis to strategic alliances. Alliances will allow us both to learn from and to influence the thinking and spending of other international actors; and they will allow us to shape what we do into a broader picture.

WHO is the lead agency in health. But we can lead more effectively when we link up with others and agree on a division of labour and on ground rules for conducting our relationships. In this way we can create real partnerships for the attainment of tangible health outcomes.

WHO is in an ideal position to play a pivotal role in sector-wide approaches – and in several countries it is already doing so. Agencies, development banks and Member States are coming to realize the disadvantages of traditional development projects. They recognize, as we do, that sectoral approaches offer a way of supporting health development that strengthens national ownership and helps to build sustainable national systems.

Our thinking on sector-wide approaches is at an early stage. There are no blueprints to show how they should be organized. But we will actively promote cooperation and joint efforts with a number of our partners – in the United Nations family, civil society and the private sector. We will do so among agencies and in our country work. Here are some of the partnerships we have been working to strengthen:

- We have worked energetically during our year as chair of the cosponsors of UNAIDS, supporting the work of achieving more common programme and budget planning.
- We have initiated a closer working relationship with the World Bank – not only on the Roll Back Malaria project and the Tobacco Free Initiative, but also by engaging in a deeper dialogue on policy issues, including in the follow-up of the Comprehensive Development Framework put forward by the President of the Bank. We are likewise beginning to intensify our efforts with the regional development banks.
- We have initiated common analyses with the International Monetary Fund. We will share with the IMF our knowledge of the health sector, working with them in seeking to avoid the harm that can occur to the social sectors during economic adjustments to financial crises.
- We have developed working relations with the World Trade Organization. In addition to contacts between our experts, I will be meeting the Director-General of WTO twice a

year on a prepared agenda. We need to interact better with WTO to make sure that the health dimension of trade and globalization is considered before and during – and not only after – complex negotiations.

- We are strengthening our work with the Organization of African Unity by upgrading our presence in Addis Ababa.
- We are updating and expanding our working relations with the European Union, an increasingly important partner in health, not only in Europe but beyond.
- We need to work with our United Nations partners to help refine the purpose of the UN Development Assistance Framework process, and develop a clear vision of how closer coordination will be expressed in individual countries. Ideally, this will mean moving towards the development of common policy positions on key sectoral issues, and drawing other development partners into the process.
- In addition to governmental and intergovernmental partners, we are making progress in building partnerships with nongovernmental organizations and the private sector. We have had a number of round table meetings with industry. We are working closely with the Global Forum on Health Research in their efforts to catalyze greater public and private sector involvement in developing new products of relevance to the poor. The initial focus is on a public/private partnership to produce a new generation of anti-malarial drugs.

REPOSITIONING WHO FOR THE 21ST CENTURY

Helping to meet the health challenges facing the world through effectively implementing our strategic themes requires changes in WHO. Much of my work in the past ten months, and that of my colleagues, has attempted to reposition WHO internally to respond better to external needs and demands. The key objectives we identified for structural change at headquarters have either been reached or we are very close to reaching them.

The structure is flatter, and staff report to a competent and clearly mandated senior management with clear priorities. There is more transparency through more open decision-making in a new Cabinet form of governance, where heads of the nine clusters of departments meet on a weekly basis. We are moving with determination towards gender parity. We have initiated a process of staff rotation and mobility. There is a new dialogue with staff.

Some reforms need time. We wish to see the number of senior positions come down – and they will. But in getting there we are fully respecting contracts and previous commitments. We have reduced administrative costs. And we will go further. It is my ambition to see to it that our administrative and programme reviews identify further scope for redirection of funds from administrative to technical activities.

Having spent ten months at WHO I feel I can say this: staff serving the United Nations are hard-working people, often accepting workloads that many national civil servants would turn down. These staff constitute our ultimate resource. Providing them with the tools, skills and mandates to work effectively is the objective of our personnel policies, and I believe we are beginning to see results.

Our work in this initial phase is about WHO renewal, and I wish to see this penetrate everything we do: safeguarding what works, drawing on experience and knowledge, but looking ahead to serve a world in dramatic change. The challenge now is to work better and focus our efforts on where the return in health gains is greatest. In this we intend to draw more heavily on the wisdom and experience of the WHO Executive Board and to create a shared vision and sense of direction with our country representatives. In February, for the first time ever, we brought together all our country representatives to introduce them to the change process and to learn from their experiences.

With structural changes at headquarters behind us, we are now engaging closely with the regions. The regional offices are a major strength of WHO. Many United Nations agencies are struggling to decentralize. WHO has already done it. Now the task is to make the whole Organization pull together, pursuing a shared corporate strategy. Our target is "One WHO" – aiming to make our contribution to better health outcomes for the populations we are here to serve, through our own work and through our work in partnerships with others.

The purpose of our work is to improve people's lives, reduce the burdens of disease and poverty, and provide access to responsive health care for all. We must never lose this vision. Thanks to the support of our Member States and the commitment of our staff, we are beginning to see results on the ground. In my next message I look forward to reporting on how we have made a difference and on the measurable improvements that have been achieved as we move into a new century.

Gro Harlem Brundtland
Geneva
May 1999

PART ONE

MAKING A DIFFERENCE IN PEOPLE'S LIVES:
Achievements and Challenges

Part One begins, in Chapter 1, by reviewing the dramatic decline in mortality in the 20th century. Income growth and improved educational levels – and consequent improvements in food intake and sanitation – have accounted for part of the mortality decline; but access to new knowledge, drugs and vaccines appears to have been substantially more important. The decline in mortality has had far-reaching consequences for every aspect of life: fertility began a rapid decline, populations are ageing and better health has contributed to the wide diffusion of rapid economic growth.

Chapter 2 then turns to the double burden of disease that health systems of the 21st century must address. One element of the double burden results, ironically, from the successes of the 20th century: as a consequence of the ageing of populations, epidemics of noncommunicable disease and injury now drive the demand for health resources. Meanwhile, not everyone has shared the benefits of better health. Large inequalities persist in well-off countries, and as many as a billion people still suffer heavily from conditions that are virtually unseen among the non-poor. This unfinished agenda – the second element of the double burden – is described, and the chapter shows that relatively inexpensive tools exist for dealing with these problems.

1

HEALTH AND DEVELOPMENT

IN THE 20TH CENTURY

*T*he 20th century has seen a global transformation in human health unmatched in history. The magnitude of this transformation can be illustrated by looking at the example of Chile. By the mid-1990s, Chile had a per capita income of about US$ 4000 (adjusted for purchasing power of currency), i.e. it had a high average standard of living, with an income level sufficient to provide its people with more than adequate food, shelter and sanitation. Yet Chilean women today have a life expectancy of 79 years – perhaps 25 years more than women in a country with a similar income level in 1900 (and 46 years more than Chilean women had in the early 1900s). This chapter briefly describes this 20th century revolution in human health, then examines both its profound consequences for human demography and its contribution to the worldwide diffusion of rapid economic growth.

THE 20TH CENTURY REVOLUTION IN HUMAN HEALTH

The steady improvement in life expectancy that began in Europe in the late 1900s continued virtually without interruption throughout the 20th century. In England and Wales for example, life expectancy was around 40 years in the late 19th century; but by early in the 20th century it had risen to almost 50 years. Other countries experienced similar take-off periods. In Europe these mostly occurred in the late 19th or early 20th century.

Economic historians and demographers debate the genesis of these increases in life expectancy, but the increases appear to be at least partially linked to the economic changes resulting from the agricultural and industrial revolutions. One aspect of economic change – urbanization – actually affected health adversely by exposing an increasing proportion of the population to crowded conditions, thereby facilitating the spread of infection. Somewhat more than counterbalancing this effect, though, were increases in nutrient intake and improvements in sanitation and water supply resulting from higher income levels *(1)*. Better health and nutritional status were both a result and a cause of income growth. Although northern Europeans had began immunizing against smallpox by early in the 19th century, this was exceptional, and other specific knowledge and tools for improving health probably played only a limited role in the minor health improvements of the 19th century *(2)*. In contrast, the 20th century health revolution appears to have resulted far more substantially from the generation and application of new knowledge.

Mortality rates in European countries continued their decline in the 20th century, and by the second half of the century this mortality revolution had spread to the rest of the world. The 20th century global revolution in health transformed – and is transforming – not only the quality of individual lives, but also the demography of populations. These changed health and demographic circumstances have themselves contributed to wide diffusion of economic growth. This chapter overviews the health revolution and its demographic and economic consequences, as well as looking at why it occurred. Chapter 2 then turns to the epidemiological consequences of the health revolution that result from ageing populations, and describes how the incompleteness of the health revolution has left perhaps a billion people behind. Addressing this "double burden" is perhaps the central issue for health policy for the 21st century.

THE PRECIPITOUS DECLINE IN MORTALITY

Whereas life expectancy in England and Wales varied around an average of 40 years during the two centuries prior to 1870, in the subsequent 125 years it almost doubled. Other countries shared this pattern of improvement in the 20th century, as Table 1.1 shows.

Chile, to continue with the example, provides an interesting and well-documented case where the take-off in life expectancy occurred well within this century. The life expectancy at birth for a Chilean female in 1910 was 33 years. Today her life expectancy would be 78 years, an increase of a remarkable 45 years. How has that made a difference in the lives of Chilean women? Figure 1.1 quantifies one obvious dimension of change: the probability that a Chilean female would die before her fifth birthday has declined from 36% to 1.9%. Less obvious, perhaps, is that throughout middle life death rates are far lower; she is now much less likely to die as a young adult from tuberculosis or in child-

Table 1.1 Life expectancy at birth, selected countries, around 1910 and in 1998

Country	Around 1910		1998	
	Males	Females	Males	Females
Australia	56	60	75	81
Chile	29	33	72	78
England and Wales	49	53	75	80
Italy	46	47	75	81
Japan	43	43	77	83
New Zealand[a]	60	63	74	80
Norway	56	59	75	81
Sweden	57	59	76	81
United States[b]	49	53	73	80

[a] Excluding Maoris.
[b] Registration states only; includes District of Columbia.

Sources: 1910 data: **Preston SH, Keyfitz N, Schoen R**. *Causes of death: Life tables for national populations.* New York. and London, Seminar Press, 1972. For Australia: **Cumpston JHL (Lewis MJ ed.)** *Health and disease in Australia: A history.* Department of Community Services and Health, Canberra, AGPS, 1989.

1998 data: **United Nations Population Division.** *World population prospects: The 1998 revision.* New York, United Nations, 1998.

Figure 1.1 Age distribution of deaths in Chile, females, 1909 and 1999 cohorts

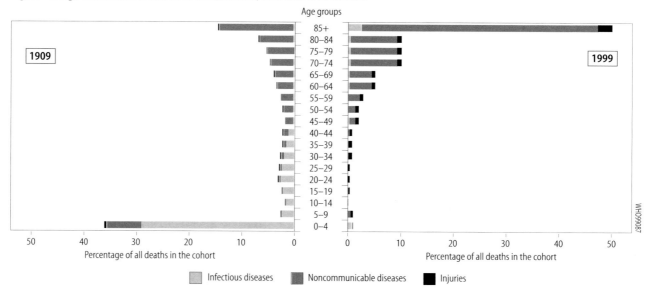

birth, or in middle age from cancer. Mirroring this mortality reduction – but less easily quantified – are marked changes in her health-related quality of life. She will spend less time in pregnancy and child-rearing. From an average of about 5.3 children at mid-century, Chilean women's fertility has dropped to its current level of 2.3 – barely above replacement level. She will have fewer infections, less anaemia, greater strength and stature, and a quicker mind. Her life is not only much longer, it is much healthier as well.

While Chile's progress in this century has been exceptional, most low and middle income countries have undergone (or are undergoing) a similar transformation of health and mortality levels. Recent exceptions to these favourable trends occur in AIDS-ravaged parts of Africa and, for a variety of reasons, among adult males in central and eastern Europe.

DEMOGRAPHIC TRANSITION

Although mortality declines have typically led to increases in population growth rates, these increases prove temporary. Fertility decline accompanies or soon follows mortality decline, bringing growth rates back to low levels. Figure 1.2 shows a half century of decline, for each WHO Region, in total fertility rate (TFR) – the expected number of children a woman would bear at the prevailing age-specific fertility rates. A TFR of a little over 2 represents a replacement level of fertility, i.e. a level that if maintained in the long run would result neither in population growth nor decline.

At mid-century, fertility rates were extremely high in most countries of the world (with the exception of the high income countries). TFRs of 6 were not uncommon. Figure 1.2 shows that every region except Africa has experienced sharp declines in fertility. And evidence is mounting that the decline in Africa has now commenced.

Declining birth rates lead to stabilization in the size of the youngest age cohorts. Over time these youths become middle-aged, while the younger cohorts remain about the same size. Figure 1.3 provides a further example of change, with data illustrating the population age distributions (pyramids) in WHO's South-East Asia Region for 1950, 2000 and 2050. After the rapid decline in fertility, age distributions change, but only slowly. If the South-East Asia Region's TFR remains at 2.9, its average population age will continue increasing for decades to come.

The world today is perhaps somewhat past the halfway point of a two-century period during which the demographic characteristics of the human population will have been totally transformed. This transformation (or demographic transition) entails a move from very high birth and death rates to low ones; a move from initially low population growth rates through a period of high rates and a vast increase in total population then back to low or zero growth rates; and a move from an age distribution with numerous young and few elderly to one with nearly equal numbers in most age groups. Enormous social, economic and epidemiological changes follow the demographic transition, which is itself a consequence of the still-ongoing revolution in mortality. Chapter 2 will point to the epidemiological consequences of the demographic transition and the concluding section of this chapter will outline possible economic consequences. This report simply notes the great importance of these changes, rather than discussing them in any detail.

Figure 1.2 Declines in fertility by WHO Region, 1950 and 1998

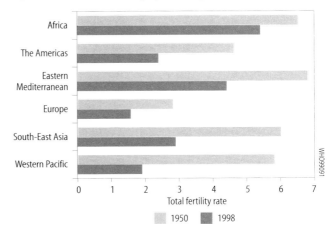

Source: **United Nations Population Division.** *World population prospects: The 1998 revision.* New York, United Nations, 1998.

Figure 1.3 **Distribution of the population of the South-East Asia Region, by age and sex, 1950, 2000 and 2050**

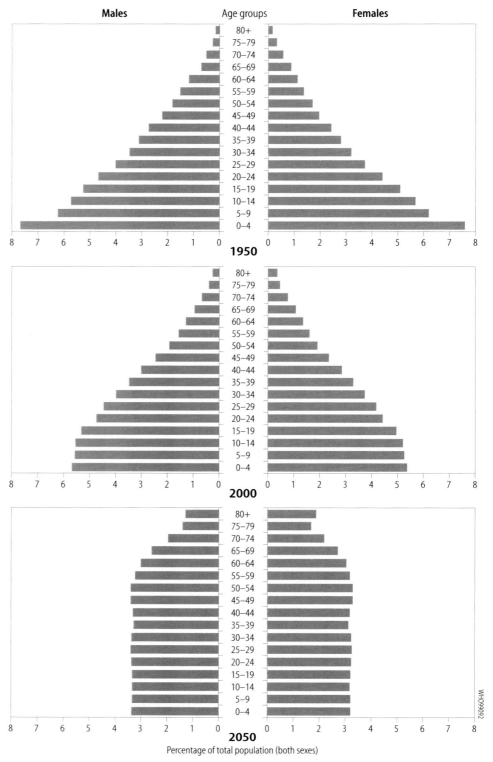

Source: **United Nations Population Division.** *World population prospects: The 1998 revision.* New York, United Nations, 1998.

SOURCES OF MORTALITY DECLINE

Income improvements can lead to mortality reductions, and numerous studies have attempted to quantify this effect. Analyses undertaken as background to this report, for example, assessed for all countries the effects of national income on health outcomes during the period 1952–1992. Figure 1.4 shows results from this analysis in curves relating the infant mortality rate (IMR) to gross domestic product (GDP) per capita (adjusted for purchasing power). Income increases do indeed correlate with mortality declines and there are good reasons to believe that the relation is causal in both directions.

How much of the remarkable decline in infant mortality rates has resulted from income growth during that period? The upper curve shows the income–mortality relation in 1952 and the lower one, for 1992, shows how much lower mortality rates had become by then for any given level of income. Figure 1.4 suggests that however important income growth may be, *the changing relation between mortality and other factors (e.g. access to health technology) is likely to be more important*. Between 1952 and 1992, for example, per capita income increased by about two thirds, on average, across the countries included in the analysis – from about $1530 to $2560. The upper curve in Figure 1.4 shows that had the income–mortality relation remained as it was in 1952, the IMR would have declined from 144 to 116. In fact it declined to only 55.

Table 1.2 reports the results of an attempt to quantify the relative importance of key determinants of mortality reduction. It draws on a statistical assessment of how the relation has changed over time between various health indicators and both income levels and average educational levels (of adult females). The table reflects a decomposition of the causes of improvement in health into three components: increases in average income levels; improvements in average educational levels; and a favourable shift in the underlying curve. This favourable shift is ascribed to the generation

Table 1.2 Sources of mortality reduction, 1960–1990

Reduction	Percentage contribution of gains in		
	Income	Educational level of adult females	Generation and utilization of new knowledge
Under-5 mortality rate	17	38	45
Female adult mortality rate	20	41	39
Male adult mortality rate	25	27	49
Female life expectancy at birth	19	32	49
Male life expectancy at birth	20	30	50
Total fertility rate	12	58	29

Note: The results are based on analysis of data from 115 low and middle income countries.

Source: **Wang J et al**. *Measuring country performance on health: Selected indicators for 115 countries*. Washington DC, The World Bank, 1999 (Human Development Network, Health, Nutrition and Population Series).

Figure 1.4 The role of improvements in income in reducing infant mortality rates

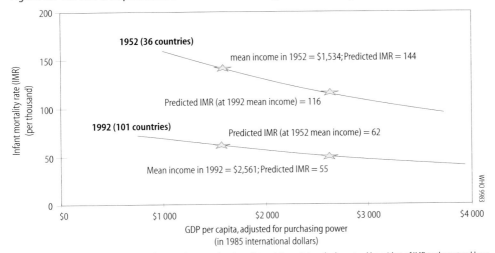

Note: Results are based on a cross-sectional time-series regression that relates, at 5-year intervals, the natural logarithm of IMR to the natural logarithm of income, the square of the natural logarithm of income and indicator variables for time. Data sources are the same as for Annex Table 6.

and application of new knowledge. Other indicators of social welfare show a similarly modest relation to income growth along with favourable time trends at any given level of income (3). Much research remains to be done, however, in order to achieve a complete understanding of why the income–health relation has improved so much. Typically, half the gains in health between 1952 and 1992 result from access to better technology. The remaining gains result from movement along the curve (income improvements and, more importantly, better education). Figure 1.4 (which does not control for education changes) illustrates the magnitude of the effect of moving along the curve relative to shifts in the curve (4,5). Higher levels of income and education affect health through a variety of mechanisms, often involving many sectors of the economy. Box 1.1 outlines the main multisectoral determinants of health.

The historical evidence points in the same direction. In some countries, many decades of economic growth saw no change in health status (for example, England and Wales); in Sweden the take-off in health occurred at about the same time as in Britain but economic growth began three-quarters of a century later; and in India the take-off in life expectancy preceded that for economic growth (2).

Shifting the curve and *moving along the curve* are, then, both sources of improvements in health. Some countries lie far above the curve, i.e. their mortality rates are much higher than would be predicted by their income. For these countries, *joining the curve* may be the quickest way to improve health. Chapter 2 will illustrate the extent to which some of the world's most populous countries could make great health gains by joining the curve.

What conclusions can be drawn from this analysis? First and foremost, it is clear that

---

Box 1.1 The multisectoral determinants of health

Hungry children easily acquire diseases, and easily die from the diseases they do acquire. Dwellings without sanitation provide fertile environments for transmission of intestinal infections. Air dense with particulates or acids destroys lungs, and lives. Hopeless life circumstances thrust young girls (and boys) into prostitution with its attendant risks of violence and sexually transmitted diseases, including HIV/AIDS. Manufacturers of tobacco and alcohol profit enormously from advertising and promotion that spreads addiction. Rapid growth in vehicular traffic – often with untrained drivers on unsafe roads – generates a rising toll of injury. Poorly designed irrigation projects create breeding grounds for vectors of disease. The list could be much extended, and it could be rephrased in terms of factors favorable to health, but the point is clear: determinants of health are truly multisectoral.

An assessment commissioned for WHO's 1997 Ad Hoc Committee on Health Research estimated the percentage of deaths, by region and globally, associated with each of ten risk factors. It concluded that the following risks contributed to global mortality in 1990:

- tobacco use – 6.0%;
- hypertension – 5.8%;
- inadequate water and sanitation – 5.3%.
- risky sexual activity – 2.2%;
- alcohol use – 1.5%;

Underlying most specific risks are more general determinants of health – income and education levels. The effects of income and education operate for the most part through influencing risk (and being able to utilize health services effectively). For example, poorer societies may forego expensive mechanisms for cleaning polluted air or water from factories, and poorer households lack the resources to purchase indoor sanitation or piped water. Poorly educated individuals may fail to observe basic hygiene or neglect appropriate weaning practices for their children; and they are increasingly the population that smokes. The effects of education and income are indeed real and quantitatively important, even though only about half of health improvements in developing countries in the period 1960–1990 result from these factors.

If an important fraction of ill-health results from poverty and low educational levels – or from their consequences in inadequate food or sanitation or other specific risks – then ought the task of the health professional lie principally in addressing these underlying problems? In one sense the answer is surely yes: the health community should measure the effects on health of actions outside the health sector. It should ensure that these findings are communicated, and are considered in making policy choices. The magnitude of the demonstrated effect of girls' education on health and fertility outcomes, for example, provides a powerful argument for investing in extension of educational access to girls.

But the health community has limited capacity for direct action outside the health sector – and limited credibility. It will make more of a difference if it focuses its energy, expertise and resources on ensuring that health systems efficiently deliver the powerful interventions provided by modern science.

Source: *Investing in health research and development. Report of the Ad Hoc Committee on Health Research Relating to Future Intervention Options.* Geneva, World Health Organization, 1996 (document WHO/TDR/Gen/96.1).

health system development is a key priority. The effects of economic growth on health, while real, are relatively weak and likely to be slow in coming. Rather than waiting for movement along the curve, *countries should focus health system development on the task of joining the curve* or going beyond it to the point of best practice.

Second, in the medium to long term, shifting the curve will underpin health improvements. The high income countries now commit vast sums (over US$ 55 billion per year) to the research and development (R&D) efforts that will shift the curve favourably. But only a fraction of that amount is directed to solving the particular problems of poor and disadvantaged people. Greater R&D commitments to such problems would be likely to pay off enormously in improving health. Ensuring an adequate commitment to R&D is surely an integral element of health system development.

There is every reason to expect, then, that focused investments by health systems on specific problems of the poor can generate major short to medium term gains in health, and that investment in R&D can sustain medium to long term gains. Such gains are of immense intrinsic value. The association between income and health moreover suggests that health investments may have an economic payoff as well. Supporting evidence for this assertion is presented below. Indeed, rather than continuing to point to poverty as the root cause of ill-health, decision-makers may come to focus on the two-way relationship between poverty and ill-health, identifying the latter as one of the root causes of poverty – and one that is particularly amenable to public intervention.

HEALTH AND ECONOMIC PRODUCTIVITY

The global gains in health documented above constitute, arguably, humankind's most dramatic achievement. In our era it is *possible* for every individual to expect to live a long and substantially disease-free life. This accomplishment transcends the need for economic valuation. Health gains have intrinsic value. That said, two particular reasons exist for assessing the economic consequences of better health:

- Understanding health's economic role may help to understand the sources of another of humankind's great accomplishments of the 20th century – widespread rapid economic growth. To the extent that better health has contributed to increased growth rates, investing in health can become a tool of macroeconomic policy.
- Conquering poverty constitutes the central task for development policy at the beginning of the 21st century. Despite rapid economic growth, over a billion humans still exist in absolute, degrading poverty. Because ill-health traps people in poverty, sustained investment in the health of the poor could provide a policy lever for alleviating persistent poverty.

Research has begun to provide clearer evidence of the economic benefits of improving health. But data sets underpinning the research – on characteristics of countries over time or on large numbers of households within a country at a given time – rarely permit conclusive determination of cause and effect. Conclusions drawn from the literature remain, therefore, suggestive rather than definitive. Those conclusions do, though, accord with common sense: healthier people are more productive. Health differences have played a significant role in determining why some countries have grown more rapidly than others, although technological advances and physical capital accumulation may have been more important still.

What is the evidence? This section summarizes the literature by, first, reviewing cross-country macroeconomic analyses, then by turning to microeconomic comparisons across households. It closes with a brief discussion of the multiple pathways through which better health influences economic outcomes.

MACROECONOMIC EVIDENCE

Since publication of Adam Smith's *The wealth of nations* over two centuries ago, economists have sought answers to the question of why some countries are wealthy and others poor. Why have economic growth rates differed? The main empirical tool now used to study economic growth is cross-country analysis of the relationship between economic growth (typically measured in terms of the growth rate of per capita GDP) and a range of variables believed to account for why growth rates differ *(6,7)*. Among the factors being explored are: levels and patterns of educational attainment (schooling); population growth, density and age structure; natural resource abundance; personal and government saving (investment rates); physical capital stock; economic policy, for example, the degree of trade openness; the quality of public institutions; and geography, for example, the location and climate of a country.

Recent research has added several specific health indicators to these factors, and looked at the links between them and economic growth. There are direct links between economic performance and health indicators such as life expectancy. Some variables, such as geography and demography, indirectly link health with economic growth. Geography, particularly tropical location, is highly correlated with disease burden, which in turn affects economic performance *(8)*. Demography, on the other hand, is determined in part by health status, and has a direct effect on economic growth through the age structure of the population, in particular the ratio of the working age to the total population.

A major result to emerge from recent research is that survival rates or life expectancy are powerful predictors of income levels or of subsequent economic growth. The studies consistently find a strong effect of health on economic levels or growth rates. Interestingly, economic historians have concluded that perhaps 30% of the estimated per capita growth rate in Britain between 1780 and 1979 was a result of improvement in health and nutritional status *(9)*. That figure lies within the range of estimates produced by cross-country studies using data from the last 30 or 40 years *(10)*.

Health improvements also influence economic growth through their impact on demography. For example, in the 1940s, rapid improvements in health in East Asia provided a catalyst for a demographic transition there. An initial decline in infant and child mortality swelled the youth population, and somewhat later prompted a fall in fertility rates. These asynchronous changes in mortality and fertility, which comprise the first phase of the demographic transition, substantially altered East Asia's age distribution. After a time lag, the working-age population began growing much faster than the young dependent population, temporarily creating a disproportionately high percentage of working-age adults. This bulge in the age structure of the population created an opportunity for increased rates of economic growth. By introducing these demographic considerations into an empirical model of economic growth, analyses undertaken for the Asian Development Bank (ADB) were able to show that East Asia's changing demography can explain perhaps a third to half the economic "miracle" experienced between 1965 and 1990 *(11,12)*.

The ADB study cautions that although a "demographic gift" provides an opportunity for increasing prosperity, it by no means guarantees such results. East Asia's growth rates were achieved because government and the private sector were able to mobilize this burgeoning work force by successfully managing other economic opportunities. Adopting new industrial technologies, investing in basic education and exploiting global markets allowed East

Asia to realize the economic growth potential created by the demographic transition. The next phase for East Asia will involve less favourable dependency ratios consequent to population ageing. In contrast, both South Asia and Africa are now entering the period when demographic factors can enhance growth prospects. Box 1.2 describes ongoing work assessing linkages between health and income in the Americas.

Analysts are extending this research in several ways. One line of work, analysing the effects of climate on income, concludes that countries in tropical regions suffer important disadvantages relative to those in temperate zones. In addition to the effects of climate and geography on soil quality, this work suggests that an important causal mechanism through which this effect operates is the interaction of tropical climates and tropical diseases, particularly malaria which can have a significant cost in terms of economic performance *(8)*. Another line of analysis suggests that the interaction of exogenous demographic changes with human and physical capital development can lead to a virtuous cycle of growth, enabling a country to break free of a poverty trap *(13)*.

MICROECONOMIC ANALYSIS

Unlike macroeconomic studies that compare the performance of countries over time, microeconomic analyses study the link between health and the income of households and individuals. Until recently, much of the microeconomic literature has dealt with the impact of education and training on labour outcomes. Recent individual and household level studies have, however, paid more attention to health (particularly nutritional aspects of health) and are reaching increasingly consistent findings *(14)*.

Several examples provide an indication of the results of this research. In Indonesia, men with anaemia were found to be 20% less productive than men without it. In one of the few experimental studies in the literature, the anaemic men were randomly assigned to one of two groups in a clinical trial – they received either an iron supplement or a placebo. Those who were initially anaemic and received the iron treatment increased their productivity nearly to the levels of non-anaemic workers, and the productivity gains were large when weighed against the costs of treatment. Thus the effects of improved health were found to be greatest for the most vulnerable, that is, the poorest and those with the least education. Box 1.3 provides more detail on another study, also from Indonesia and also involving an

---

Box 1.2 Assessment of the links between health and productivity: a PAHO initiative

In recent years, WHO Member States in the Region of the Americas have expressed interest in improving the understanding of linkages between investments in health, economic growth and poverty reduction. In response, a joint PAHO/Inter-American Development Bank/UNECLAC study has been initiated aiming at elucidating relations between investments in health, economic growth and household productivity. Preliminary data from Latin American and Caribbean countries show that growth in GDP is statistically associated with life expectancy, as has been found in other studies for a wider sample of countries. Life expectancy at birth alone is one of the strongest explanatory variables of growth in GDP.

Estimates based on data from Mexico throw some light on the timeframe in which health affects economic indicators. High life expectancy at birth for males and females has an economic impact 0–5 years later. The impact of male life expectancy on the economy is greater than that of female life expectancy, probably because of the higher level of economic activity among males. The results suggest that for any additional year of life expectancy there will be an additional 1% increase in GDP 15 years later. Similar findings were observed for schooling. In this case, the correlation between female life expectancy and schooling is greater than that for male life expectancy, probably because of the larger role that women play in child-rearing.

This work drew the implication for economic policy that the relationship between health improvement variables and economic growth is sufficiently significant in the long term to justify sustained national commitment to investing in health. Continued work by PAHO – and its collaborators – should further elucidate these linkages at both the household level and the national level.

Contributed by the WHO Regional Office for the Americas/Pan American Health Organization.

intervention. Here the intervention (introduction of user fees) resulted in lower levels of nutritional status and productivity among those initially poor *(15)*.

A careful statistical analysis of the effects of illness on wages and labour supply in Côte d'Ivoire and Ghana found that wages were significantly lower, in both countries, for each day of disability. Ill-health in the form of disability, in these poor communities, contributed to their continuing poverty *(16)*.

At the household level, it is also possible to measure directly the economic burden created by particular diseases. Tuberculosis provides a relevant example. The economic costs of tuberculosis are made up of two main elements. First, there are the direct costs of prevention and treatment (drugs, health care provider fees, transport, and costs of subsistence at a health centre). Second, there are the indirect costs of labour time lost because of illness. Given these two components of cost, there are several ways in which tuberculosis affects economic outcomes. Tuberculosis-related morbidity directly increases household and public sector expenditures. It reduces labour inputs and can reduce human capital as a result of declines in school attendance. In a case study of costs of improving tuberculosis control in Thailand in 1995, the cost of treatment was estimated to be US$ 343 per case. The researchers also estimated the total indirect cost of lost productivity in Thailand as a result of morbidity associated with treated and untreated cases of tuberculosis, amounting to $57 million.

PATHWAYS OF INFLUENCE

Delineating potential pathways of influence sheds light on health's role within the larger web of determinants of income levels and growth rates. A paper presented to the World Health Assembly in 1952 foreshadowed much of the current work on understanding these pathways *(17)*.

Box 1.3 User fees, health outcomes and labour force participation in Indonesia: a two-year study

In an intervention study in Indonesia – the Indonesian Resource Mobilization Study (IRMS) – the effect of changes in prices of publicly provided health services on labour force participation was examined. In the experiment, user fees at public health centres were raised in randomly selected test districts, while fees were held constant (in real terms) in neighbouring control districts. A baseline household survey was conducted at the end of 1991, prior to the intervention, and the same households, evenly divided between those that were subjected to the fee increase and those that were not, were surveyed again two years later. The experiment involved 6000 households in several districts in each of two provinces. One of the provinces was well-to-do and one

was poor. Equal numbers of control and test households were selected from each province.

Use of health care declined in test areas, relative to controls, as did some health status indicators. Using self-reports about limitations in their ability to perform activities of daily living – such as walking 5 kilometres, carrying a heavy load 20 metres, or having spent a day in bed in the previous month – the follow-up study in 1993 showed that the great majority of those where prices had been raised showed at least some ill effects. In IRMS, higher prices are associated with greater difficulty walking 5 kms, more limitations on daily activities and more days spent in bed. For example, both men and women in the test districts reported having had to spend an average of a third of a day in bed more

than the control group because of illness. But the effects were much greater among the poor, among men over 40, and among women in households with low economic and educational status. Men in the bottom quartile of per capita income in the test areas reported losing almost a full day more of activity compared to the control group.

Moreover, the follow-up study showed significant declines in labour force participation in the test area among the more vulnerable groups. Men in the over 40 age group had a slight tendency to drop out of the labour market in the test area. Among all women in the survey, both in the control and test groups, labour force participation dropped from 50% to 46% between 1991 and 1993, but there was a 7.3 percentage point dif-

ference between those in the test and control groups, to the disadvantage of those paying higher health fees. In the test districts, labour force participation for women with no education fell 14%. Women over 40 were also likely to have high dropout rates from the labour market in the areas where health costs had gone up.

Wage rates for men were also affected. While on average both test and control groups increased their nominal wages by 30% in the two years, the increase came 15% sooner in the control areas. The comparative slippage in the test areas was particularly great for older workers, whose health is presumably a greater factor in their work performance.

Source: **Dow WH et al.** *Health care prices, health and labor outcomes: Experimental evidence.* Santa Monica CA, RAND, 1997 (unpublished paper).

There is evidence that adult health depends in part on child health and itself directly influences labour productivity. Per capita income is defined as the level of income divided by total population. Clearly, the total population consists of economic dependents as well as the economically active. Improved adult health will improve the dependency ratio both by reducing mortality among the economically active and by reducing premature retirement that results from illness *(18)*, and this ratio changes as a result of demographic transition (see Figure 1.5, upper part). In Jamaica, for example, individuals with chronic disease were found to be more likely to retire than those who are healthy *(19)*. Better adult health directly affects productivity by increasing work output and reducing absenteeism. Less obviously, geographically specific diseases – onchocerciasis (river blindness) in West Africa is an example – deny communities access to valuable land or productive resources. And high levels of illness in a community may weaken links to the global economy *(20)* – links that through the movement of ideas, goods and capital help create the conditions for more rapid growth (see Figure 1.5, lower part).

Investments both in physical capital and in education underpin labour productivity. A rapidly growing literature documents the effects of ill-health on children's enrolment, learning and attendance rates in school. Many of the conditions affecting schoolchildren (e.g. intestinal worm infections and micronutrient deficiencies) respond to inexpensive but effective interventions. Recent studies in the psychological literature point to steady, long-term gains during the 20th century in the general intellectual ability of the populations of the high income countries (where data were available to generate trends). One suggested determinant of this trend lies in improved health and nutritional status *(21)*.

The ADB's studies on Asia point strongly to the effect of better health on capital formation. Expectations of a longer life appear to stimulate savings.

Economists should never forget the intrinsic value of health – or that today's health systems have the tools to vastly improve the welfare of the poor at modest cost. But neither should health professionals forget an important message for presidents and finance ministers: investing in health accelerates economic growth and is one of the very few viable approaches to rolling back poverty.

Figure 1.5 Links between health and income

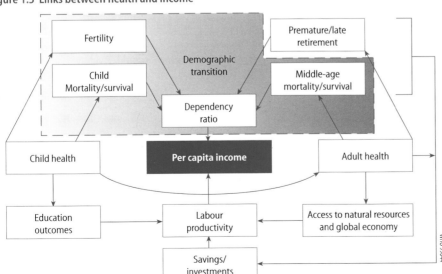

REFERENCES

1. **McKeown T.** *The role of medicine: Dream, mirage or nemesis.* London, Nuffield Provincial Hospitals Trust, 1976.

2. **Easterlin RA.** *How beneficient is the market? A look at the modern history of mortality.* Los Angeles, University of Southern California, 1998 (unpublished paper).

3. **Easterly W.** *Life during growth.* Washington DC, The World Bank, 1998 (unpublished paper).

4. **Preston SH.** The changing relation between mortality and level of economic development. *Population studies,* 1975, **29**: 213–248.

5. **Preston SH.** Causes and consequences of mortality declines in less developed countries in the 20th century. In: **Easterlin RA** (ed). *Population and economic change in developing countries.* Chicago, University of Chicago Press, 1980: 289– 341.

6. **Barro RJ.** *Determinants of economic growth: A cross-country empirical study.* Cambridge MA, The MIT Press, 1997.

7. **Sachs JD, Werner AM.** Fundamental sources of long-term growth. *American economic review,* 1997, **87**: 184–188.

8. **Gallup JL, Sachs JD, Mellinger AD.** *Geography and economic development.* Cambridge MA, Harvard Institute for International Development, 1998.

9. **Fogel RW.** New findings on secular trends in nutrition and mortality: some implications for population theory. In: **Rosenzweig MR, Stark O** (eds). *Handbook of population and family economics, Vol.1A.* Amsterdam, Elsevier Science, 1997: 433–481.

10. **Jamison DT, Lau LJ, Wang J.** Health's contribution to economic growth, 1965-90. In: *Health, health policy and economic outcomes.* Geneva, WHO Director-General's Transition Team, 1998 (Health and Development Satellite, Final Report): 61–80.

11. **Asian Development Bank.** *Emerging Asia.* Manila, Asian Development Bank, 1997.

12. **Bloom DE, Williamson JG.** Demographic transitions and economic miracles in emerging Asia. *The World Bank economic review,* 1998, **12**(3): 419–455.

13. **Bloom DE, Canning D, Malaney P.** *Population dynamics and economic growth.* Cambridge MA, Harvard Institute for International Development, 1998.

14. **Strauss J, Thomas D.** Health, nutrition and economic development. *Journal of economic literature,* 1998 **XXXVI**: 766–817.

15. **Dow WH et al.** *Health care prices, health and labor outcomes: Experimental evidence.* Santa Monica CA, RAND, 1997 (unpublished paper).

16. **Schultz TP, Tansel A.** Wage and labor supply effects of illness in Côte d'Ivoire and Ghana: instrumental variable estimates for days disabled. *Journal of development economics,* 1997, **53**: 251–286.

17. **Myrdal G.** Economic aspects of health. *Chronicle of the World Health Organization,* 1952, **6**: 203–218.

18. **Dwyer DS, Mitchell OS.** Health problems as determinants of retirement: are self-rated measures endogenous? *Journal of health economics,* 1999, **18**: 173–193.

19. **Handa S, Neitzert M.** *Chronic illness and retirement in Jamaica.* Washington DC, The World Bank, 1998 (Living Standards Measurement Study, Working Paper No.131).

20. **Radelet S, Sachs J, Lee JW.** *Economic growth in Asia.* Cambridge MA, Harvard Institute for International Development, 1997 (Development Discussion Paper No.609).

21. **Neisser V** (ed). *The rising curve: Long-term gains in IQ and related measures.* Washington DC, The American Psychological Association, 1998.

2

THE DOUBLE BURDEN:
EMERGING EPIDEMICS
AND PERSISTENT PROBLEMS

*T*he 20th century revolution in health – and the consequent demographic transition – lead inexorably to major changes in the pattern of disease. This *epidemiological* transition results in a major shift in causes of death and disability from infectious diseases to noncommunicable diseases *(1)*.

As a result of the epidemiological transition, to continue the example of Chile presented in Chapter 1, the distribution of causes of death in 1999 differs markedly from the distribution of causes of death in 1909, as shown in Figure 2.1 *(2)*. Not only have the major causes of death changed, but the average age of death has been steadily rising. The resulting new epidemics of noncommunicable disease and injuries challenge the finances and capacities of health systems.

Despite the long list of successes in health achieved globally during the 20th century, the balance sheet is indelibly stained by the avoidable burden of disease and malnutrition that the world's disadvantaged populations continue to bear. Some analysts have characterized a world of incomplete epidemiological transition, in which epidemiologically polarized sub-populations have been left behind *(3)*. Reducing the burden of that inequality is a priority in international health. Furthermore, it can be done – the means already exist.

Figure 2.1 Distribution of deaths by cause for two cohorts from Chile, 1909 and 1999

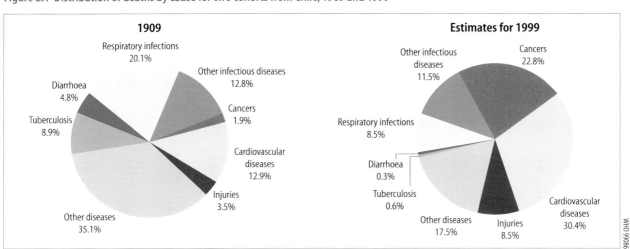

Sources: 1909 data: **Preston SH, Keyfitz N, Schoen R.** *Causes of death: Life tables for national populations.* New York and London, Seminar Press, 1972.
   1999 data: Estimates based on data from the WHO Mortality Database.

Health policy-makers in the early decades of the 21st century will thus need to address a double burden of disease: first, the emerging epidemics of noncommunicable diseases and injuries, which are becoming more prevalent in industrialized and developing countries alike, and second, some major infectious diseases which survived the 20th century – part of the unfinished health agenda. This chapter describes this double burden of disease. It points to the availability of cost-effective interventions that make it possible to complete substantially the unfinished agenda in the first decade of the 21st century. Health systems development – discussed in the next chapter – must focus on delivering these interventions for the poor.

EMERGING EPIDEMICS OF NONCOMMUNICABLE DISEASES AND INJURIES

The next two decades will see dramatic changes in the health needs of the world's populations. In the developing regions, noncommunicable diseases such as depression and heart disease are fast replacing the traditional enemies, in particular infectious diseases and malnutrition, as the leading causes of disability and premature death. Injuries, both intentional and unintentional, are also growing in importance and by 2020 could rival infectious diseases worldwide as a source of ill-health *(1)*. The rapidity of change will pose serious challenges to health care systems and force difficult decisions about the allocation of scarce resources.

To provide a valid basis for such difficult health policy decisions, there is a great need for the development of reliable and consistent data on the health status of populations worldwide. Further, as *The world health report* has argued before *(4,5)*, a new approach to measuring health status needs to be implemented, one that quantifies not merely the number of

Figure 2.2 The emerging challenges: DALYs attributable to noncommunicable diseases in low and middle income countries, estimates for 1998

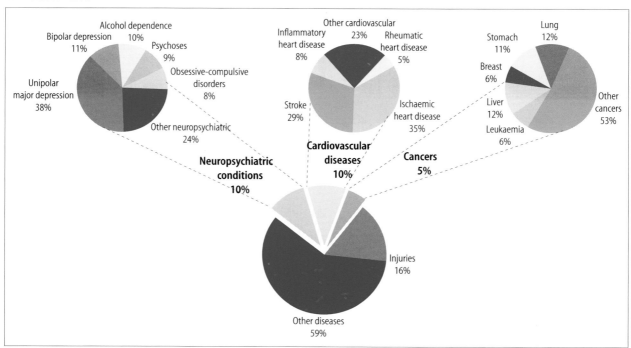

deaths but also the impact of premature death and disability on populations, and which combines them into a single unit of measurement. Several such measures have been developed in different countries, many of them being variants of the so-called Quality-Adjusted Life Year (QALY), which is principally used to measure gains from interventions. In contrast, the Disability-Adjusted Life Year (DALY) is a measure of the burden of disease.

DALYs express years of life lost to premature death and years lived with a disability, adjusted for the severity of the disability. *One DALY is one lost year of healthy life.* A "premature" death is defined as one that occurs before the age to which the dying person could have expected to survive if he or she was a member of a standardized model population with a life expectancy at birth equal to that of the world's longest-surviving population, Japan. Disease burden is, in effect, the gap between a population's actual health status and some reference status.

The initial assessment of global disease burden using DALYs was prepared in 1993 for the World Bank *(6)* in collaboration with WHO. Subsequently revisions and extensive documentation of disease burden for the year 1990 have been published *(1)*. In this report, disease burden has been quantified using "standard DALYs", calculated according to the methods described in earlier work on the burden of disease *(1)*. This report provides new estimates of disease burden for the year 1998.

NONCOMMUNICABLE DISEASES

In 1998, an estimated 43% of all DALYs globally were attributable to noncommunicable diseases. In low and middle income countries the figure was 39%, while in high income countries it was 81%. Among these diseases, the following took a particularly heavy toll (see Figure 2.2):

- neuropsychiatric conditions, accounting for 10% of the burden of disease measured in DALYs in low and middle income countries and 23% of DALYs in high income countries;
- cardiovascular diseases, responsible for 10% of DALYs in low and middle income countries and 18% of DALYs in high income countries;
- malignant neoplasms (cancers), which caused 5% of DALYs in low and middle income countries and 15% in high income countries.

One of the most surprising results of using a measure of disease burden which incorporates time lived with disability is the magnitude it ascribes to the burden of neuropsychiatric conditions. Because of the limited mortality consequences, this burden was previously underestimated. As shown in Box 2.1, a large proportion of the burden of disease resulting from neuropsychiatric conditions is attributable to unipolar major depression, which was the leading cause of disability globally in 1990. The disease burden resulting from depression is estimated to be increasing both in developing and developed regions. Alcohol use is also quantified as a major cause of disease burden, particularly for adult men. It is the leading cause of disability for men in the developed regions and the fourth leading cause in developing regions.

These findings also highlight the "hidden epidemic of cardiovascular disease" *(7)*. Within cardiovascular diseases (CVD), which collectively are responsible for about one in eight DALYs globally, ischaemic heart disease and cerebrovascular disease (stroke) are the most significant conditions. It has been estimated that ischaemic heart disease will be the largest single cause of disease burden globally by the year 2020 *(1)*. Box 2.2 discusses in more detail the nature of cardiovascular diseases in the Eastern Mediterranean Region. Substantive evidence suggests that current programmes for CVD risk factor prevention and low-cost case management offer feasible, cost-effective ways to reduce CVD mortality and disability in populations both in developed and developing countries *(8)*. Implementation of such programmes should be a priority for health policy-makers as the burden of CVD rises in all socioeconomic groups and inflicts major human and economic costs on societies.

The third largest cause of disease burden within noncommunicable conditions is cancer. Cancers are responsible for a large proportion of years of life lost and years lived with disability. Among cancers, the most significant cause of disease burden is lung cancer, which is projected to become ever more prevalent over the next few decades, if current smoking trends continue. Tobacco is a major risk factor for several other noncommunicable diseases as well. As discussed in detail in Chapter 5, tobacco control is one of the major public health priorities for the 21st century.

Noncommunicable diseases are expected to account for an increasing share of disease burden, rising from 43% in 1998 to 73% by 2020, assuming a continuation of recent downward trends in overall mortality (which have yet to be realized in China and elsewhere) *(9)*. The expected increase is likely to be particularly rapid in developing countries. In India, deaths from noncommunicable causes are projected to almost double from about 4.5 million in 1998 to about 8 million a year in 2020.

The steep projected increase in the burden of noncommunicable diseases worldwide – the epidemiological transition – is largely driven by population ageing, augmented by the rapidly increasing numbers of people who are at present exposed to tobacco and other risk factors, such as obesity, physical inactivity and heavy alcohol consumption. This increase in noncommunicable diseases induced by changes in age distribution poses significant problems. Health systems must adjust to deal effectively and efficiently with the globally chang-

---

Box 2.1 The rising burden of neuropsychiatric disorders

Disease priorities change dramatically as measurement of disease burden shifts from simple mortality indicators to indicators that incorporate disability. Neuropsychiatric conditions have been ignored for a long time as they are absent from cause of death lists. However, when disease burden measurement includes time lived with a disability, several of the neuropsychiatric disorders become leading causes of disease burden worldwide.

Annex Table 3 reports that 11% of the global burden of disease in 1998 was attributable to neuropsychiatric conditions; in high income countries, one out of every four DALYs was lost to a neuropsychiatric condition, while in low and middle income countries this group of conditions was responsible for one out of ten DALYs.

Of the ten leading causes of disease burden in young adults (in the 15–44 year age group) four were neuropsychiatric conditions. More specifically, unipolar major depression was the fourth leading cause of overall disease burden in 1990, while in adults aged 15–44 years it was the leading cause of DALYs, both in high income and in low and middle income countries. Alcohol dependence, bipolar disorder, and schizophrenia were among the leading causes of disease burden in this age group in 1998.

Great attention needs to be paid to the growing needs of populations in

Rank of selected conditions among all causes of disease burden, estimates for 1998

Disease or injury	Rank in cause-list		
	World	High income countries	Low and middle income countries
Unipolar major depression	4	2	4
Alcohol dependence	17	4	20
Bipolar disorder	18	14	19
Psychoses	22	12	24
Obsessive-compulsive disorder	28	18	27
Dementia	33	9	41
Drug dependence	41	17	45
Panic disorder	44	29	48
Epilepsy	47	34	46

Source: Annex Table 3.

the area of mental health. As shown in the table, neuropsychiatric conditions are among the leading causes of disability and burden. Psychiatric disorders are frequently a considerable drain on health resources as a consequence of being misunderstood, misdiagnosed or improperly treated. With proper budgetary planning and allocation of resources, introducing an effective mental health programme into primary health care can reduce overall health costs. Mental health care, unlike many other areas of health, does not generally demand costly technology; rather, it requires the sensitive deployment of personnel who have been properly trained in the use of relatively inexpensive drugs and psychological support skills on an outpatient basis.

ing nature of illness, and health policy-makers will be challenged to find the most cost-effective uses of their limited resources to control the rising epidemics of noncommunicable diseases. In contrast to the limited number of conditions responsible for most of the excess disease burden among the poor, policy-makers will need to develop systems capable of responding to an enormous variety of conditions as the epidemiological transition matures.

At the same time, health policy-makers will need to respond to the unexpectedly persistent inequalities in health status *within* countries. This is a problem that affects disadvantaged populations in developed and developing countries alike. Traditionally, the focus of global health policy has been on the less developed nations. Recent studies have revealed surprisingly large inequalities within developed nations, and they highlight the need for policies that focus on disadvantaged populations throughout the world. Box 2.3 summarizes some of the findings of national studies on inequalities in the USA and the UK.

INJURIES

Injuries, intentional and unintentional, are a large and neglected health problem in all regions, accounting for 16% of the global burden of disease in 1998. Figure 2.3 shows the major categories of injuries responsible for most of the burden. Road traffic accidents were the ninth leading cause of disease burden globally in 1998, fifth in the high income countries and tenth in the low and middle income countries. For adult men aged 15–44, road traffic accidents are the biggest cause of ill-health and premature death worldwide, and the second biggest in developing countries. The burden from road traffic accidents is projected to increase globally, and particularly in developing countries. In sub-Saharan Africa, partly because of the projected reduction of the burden from infectious diseases, injuries (primarily road traffic accidents, war and violence) are expected to account for a large proportion of ill-health.

Recent figures for homicides, suicides and traffic accident deaths for countries in the Americas show that these rank as the main causes of death and disability. Every year, close to 120 000 people are killed, 55 000 commit suicide, and 126 000 die in traffic accidents in the Americas *(10)*. At least 12 countries have homicide rates above 10 per 100 000 inhabitants.

Box 2.2 Cardiovascular diseases in the Eastern Mediterranean

The countries of the Eastern Mediterranean are going through an epidemiological transition, leaving many of them with the double burden of infectious and noncommunicable diseases. The ageing of the population, progressive urbanization, and changes in nutritional habits and lifestyles all contribute to the occurrence of cardiovascular diseases.

Although age-specific mortality rates are declining, the risk factors for cardiovascular diseases are more prevalent than before. Diets have a higher fat content; there are over 17 million people with diabetes and a further 17 million with impaired glucose tolerance; smoking is widespread especially among younger people; and physical activity is insufficient. Prevention has the potential to reduce mortality further.

Mortality data are inadequate in many countries of the Eastern Mediterranean, but available information shows that coronary heart disease is increasing as a cause of hospital admission and is being seen at younger ages than before. Hypertension has been reported to affect more than 20% of adults, but it is estimated that more than half of the cases are not diagnosed.

Community-based intervention programmes have been shown to be effective in promoting healthy lifestyles and reducing the incidence of cardiovascular diseases. WHO is therefore working with countries to establish pilot projects to provide information on risk factors and to promote healthy lifestyles with regard to tobacco use, diet and physical activity. Special emphasis is placed on inculcating good habits in children and adolescents. Efforts are made to involve local groups and community decision-makers, so as to mobilize the community and ensure that people are able to follow healthier lifestyles.

Contributed by the WHO Regional Office for the Eastern Mediterranean.

Violence and self-inflicted injuries (including suicide) are a major public health concern because of their increasing significance within the global disease burden. Injuries primarily affect the younger age groups and often result in disabling conditions. In higher income countries, road traffic accidents and self-inflicted injuries were among the ten leading causes of disease burden in 1998 as measured in DALYs. In less developed countries, road traffic accidents were the most significant cause of injuries, ranking eleventh among the most important causes of lost years of healthy life. War, violence and self-inflicted injuries were all among the leading twenty causes of such loss in those countries. Intentional injuries primarily affect young adults, with males in the age group of 15–34 years bearing a particularly large proportion of the burden.

Domestic violence, especially against women, is not always reflected in physical injury but may be apparent in psychological sequelae. Traditionally, violence has been classified as intentional injury. While it is clearly important to recognize violence as a cause of injury,

Figure 2.3 The emerging challenges: DALYs attributable to injuries in low and middle income countries, estimates for 1998

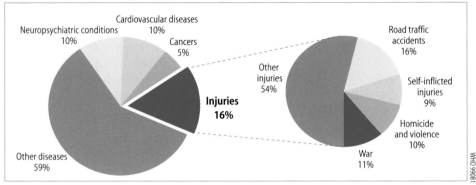

Source: Annex Table 3.

Box 2.3 Health inequalities in the USA and the UK

The use of national life expectancy at birth as a measure of health and well-being of a population places the United States among the better-off countries. National life expectancy has been rising steadily for both men and women in the last half of the century. National life expectancy is an aggregate measure and masks the remarkable variation that is observed within the nation. The results from the on-going study on the burden of disease and injury in the USA have shown that at the county level, the range in life expectancy is similar to the range observed across all countries. The range in life expect-

ancy between females in Stearns, Minnesota and males in Bennett, Jackson, Mellette, Shannon, Todd and Washabaugh counties, South Dakota, is 22.48 years. This range becomes even wider – 41.3 years – when race-specific life expectancy across counties is calculated. This difference of 41.3 years corresponds to 90% of the global range from the population with the lowest life expectancy (males in Sierra Leone) to the population with the highest (females in Japan).

The USA has been reasonably successful at reducing the inequalities in absolute terms (not relative terms) in child and adolescent mortality as com-

pared to the range in mortality observed between the established market economies and sub-Saharan Africa. On the other hand, the USA has been much less successful in reducing inequalities in adult male and to a lesser but substantial extent adult female mortality. While the focus of most public health analysis remains health conditions in children and the elderly, the largest inequalities in the USA relative to the rest of the world are found in adult male and adult female health conditions.

Large health inequalities have also been reported in the UK. Last year an independent inquiry set up by the Brit-

ish government reviewed the evidence on inequalities in health in England. The report published in November 1998 states that although average mortality rates have fallen in the last 50 years, unacceptable inequalities in health have persisted.

The report identified three crucial approaches: all policies likely to have an impact on health should be evaluated in terms of their impact on health inequalities; a high priority should be given to the health of families with children; and further steps should be taken to reduce income inequalities and improve the living standards of poor households.

Sources: **Murray CJL et al.** *US patterns of mortality by county and race: 1965--1994.* Cambridge MA, Harvard Center for Population and Development
  Studies, 1998 (US Burden of Disease and Injury Monograph Series).
  Report of the Independent Inquiry into Inequalities in Health. London, The Stationery Office, 1998.

particularly among women where the connection may not always be evident, the health consequences also need to be understood. So too does the different nature of the violence experienced by men, women and children.

Globally, injuries are responsible for one in six years lived with disability. Injuries have, nevertheless, often been a neglected area of public health policy. More attention therefore needs to be focused on dealing with the growing problem of injuries – through more comprehensive prevention, improved emergency and treatment services, and better rehabilitation.

PERSISTENT PROBLEMS OF INFECTIOUS DISEASES AND MATERNAL AND CHILD DISABILITY AND MORTALITY

Despite the extraordinary advances of the 20th century, a significant component of the burden of illness globally still remains attributable to infectious diseases, undernutrition and complications of childbirth. These conditions are primarily concentrated in the poorest countries, and within those countries they disproportionately afflict populations that are living in poverty. The residual concentration of infectious diseases afflicting the poor is truly an avoidable burden, because inexpensive and effective tools exist to deal with much of it. In fact, it mostly results from relatively few conditions.

The disproportionate share of the burden of disease on the poor is demonstrated in Table 2.1 and Figure 2.4, based on analyses reported in Annex Table 7. Within countries, the disadvantaged fare much worse as measured by several health indicators than the better-off. Those living in absolute poverty, compared with those who are not poor, are estimated to have a five times higher probability of death between birth and the age of 5 years, and a 2.5 times higher probability of death between the ages of 15 and 59 years. Overall, the poor fare worse than the better-off in society on all health indicators studied. Figure 2.4 demonstrates the distinctly different distributions across countries of health indicators for the poor and the non-poor. It clearly shows that the non-poor have a much higher overall health level than the poor.

These data illustrate another critical point. Some countries attain far better health conditions for their poor people than others. Poor children in China have less than a third of the risk of dying before their fifth birthday than comparably poor children in the United

Table 2.1 Health status of the poor versus the non-poor in selected countries, around 1990

Country	Percentage of population in absolute poverty[a]	Probability of dying per 1000				Prevalence of tuberculosis	
		between birth and age 5, females		between ages 15 and 59, females			
		Non-poor	Poor:non-poor ratio	Non-poor	Poor:non-poor ratio	Non-poor	Poor:non-poor ratio
Aggregate[b]		38	4.8	92	4.3	23	2.6
Chile	15	7	8.3	34	12.3	2	8.0
China	22	28	6.6	35	11.0	13	3.8
Ecuador	8	45	4.9	107	4.4	25	1.8
India	53	40	4.3	84	3.7	28	2.5
Kenya	50	41	3.8	131	3.8	20	2.6
Malaysia	6	10	15.0	99	5.1	13	3.2

[a] Poverty is defined as income per capita of less than or equal to $1 per day, expressed in dollars adjusted for purchasing power.
[b] The aggregate estimate refers to all countries listed in Annex Table 7.
See Explanatory Notes to the Statistical Annex for an explanation of the methods used to derive the estimates.
Source: Annex Table 7.

Republic of Tanzania. Poverty is not an insurmountable barrier to better health when policies are right. This further illustrates that much of the burden on the poor is unnecessary.

THE UNFINISHED AGENDA

The populations of developing countries and particularly the disadvantaged groups within those countries remain in the early stages of the epidemiological transition, where infectious diseases are still the major cause of death. Figure 2.5 depicts the distribution of deaths in low and middle income countries in 1998. It illustrates the five major childhood conditions which are responsible for 21% of all deaths in low and middle income countries: diarrhoea, acute respiratory infections, malaria, measles and perinatal conditions. Almost all DALYs from these five conditions occur in developing countries. Less than 1% are registered in high income countries. It is noteworthy that most of the DALYs among infants and young children are attributable to a limited number of conditions for which either preventive or curative interventions exist. This report will argue, in Chapter 3, that a priority for health systems development is to achieve effective delivery of these interventions, which are delineated below.

Immunization programmes have yielded the most significant changes in child health in the last few decades. Although some vaccines represent the most cost-effective public health intervention of all, the world does not use them enough. At least 2 million children still die each year from diseases for which vaccines are available at low cost. Similarly, for diarrhoeal disease, there exists a simple, inexpensive and effective intervention: oral rehydration therapy. Diarrhoeal diseases and pneumonia together account for a high proportion of deaths of children in developing countries. In several developing countries, therefore, diarrhoeal disease control programmes have been merged with a simplified approach, promoted by WHO, to detecting acute respiratory infections (primarily pneumonia).

In adults, maternal conditions, HIV/AIDS and tuberculosis are the three major causes of disease burden in developing regions, as depicted in Figure 2.5. Together, they accounted for 7% of all DALYs in 1998. Among maternal conditions, obstructed labour, sepsis and unsafe abortion were among the ten leading causes of death and disability among women aged 15–44 years in developing countries in 1998. The burden of maternal conditions has been hard to quantify because of the lack of reliable data. But it is a major public health problem and represents a major and unnecessary burden for which policy-makers should increasingly be held accountable.

Figure 2.4 Distribution of the probability of death, selected countries, around 1990

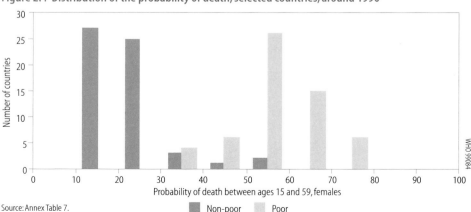

Source: Annex Table 7.   ■ Non-poor   ■ Poor

THE PERSISTING AND EVOLVING CHALLENGES

Despite the successful eradication of smallpox and the control of several infectious diseases in the 20th century, there remain some significant threats that are particularly challenging because of the changing nature of the disease pattern and the ways it manifests itself in populations. A clear example is malaria. Public health efforts in the last four decades have been remarkably effective in reducing the burden of malaria in South-East Asia and Latin America. Despite this achievement, malaria remains a major public health problem, particularly in Africa (see Annex Table 8). Malaria has been named as one of WHO's top priorities. Chapter 4 provides a detailed overview of the problem and the WHO approach to it.

Malaria, along with HIV/AIDS and tuberculosis, can be classified among a group of diseases for which control efforts are being jeopardized by microbial evolution. This problem is described in Box 2.4. Figure 2.5 demonstrates that a large proportion of the deaths occurring between the ages of 15 and 59 years in low and middle income countries can be attributed to HIV and tuberculosis. Effective and cost-effective strategies for controlling tuberculosis exist; but standard treatment regimens require six or more months of chemotherapy and rely on well-organized services to achieve high rates of adherence. The interaction of HIV and tuberculosis is also an important public health matter, as individuals who are infected with both are more likely to die from tuberculosis than from other infections. During the period of active tuberculosis infection, they may transmit the infection to previously uninfected contacts. Because HIV infection is projected to increase over the coming decade, the burden from tuberculosis may also increase unless there are energetic efforts to extend the reach of existing control measures with proven effectiveness and cost-effective-

Figure 2.5 DALYs attributable to conditions in the unfinished agenda in low and middle income countries, estimates for 1998

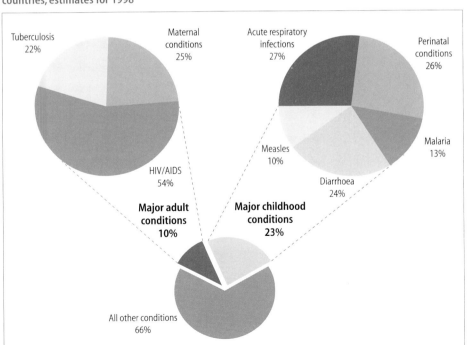

Source: Annex Table 3.

ness, as well as to invest in the development of new tools for tuberculosis control. The tuberculosis situation in the Western Pacific Region is described in Box 2.5.

The challenge posed by these persisting and evolving conditions is that tools to control them have either not been developed or, if available, are not used effectively or, in some cases, are becoming increasingly ineffective *(11)*. As examined in more detail in Box 2.4, antimicrobial resistance is a worrying phenomenon since it could have great adverse effects on the control and treatment of diseases such as pneumonia, tuberculosis and malaria. These conditions emphasize the need, as discussed further in Chapter 3, for health systems to invest in research and development strategies to come up with cost-effective tools to control the remaining threats from infectious diseases.

Increases in international air travel, trade – particularly the food trade – and tourism mean that disease-producing organisms, the deadly as well as the commonplace, can be transported rapidly from one continent to another *(4)*. This trend may threaten international public health security, although so far the consequences have remained quantitatively unimportant. To counter any such threat, the global surveillance of infectious diseases is being improved through an international information network. This should make it possible to recognize outbreaks faster.

THE AVOIDABLE BURDEN OF DISEASE

The most significant fact about the unnecessary burden is that it is concentrated on a few conditions, most of which are avoidable. There are many vaccines, drugs and clinical algorithms that if employed globally would lead to a dramatic reduction in the burden of infectious diseases. Figure 2.6 illustrates the links between infant mortality rates and per capita income in some of the most populous low and middle income countries. The countries that are above the curve in 1990 are low and middle income countries which had a higher infant mortality rate than expected, given their average income per capita. Their distance above the curve indicates potential reductions in mortality, i.e. the gains that would

---

Box 2.4 Microbial evolution – the continually changing threat of infectious disease

Resistance of disease-causing organisms to antimicrobial drugs and other agents has become a great public health concern worldwide. It is having a deadly impact on the control of diseases such as tuberculosis, malaria, cholera, dysentery and pneumonia.

Antimicrobial resistance is not a new, nor a surprising problem, but it has worsened in the last decade. All bacteria possess an inherent flexibility that enables them, sooner or later, to evolve genes that render them resistant to any antimicrobial. By killing susceptible bacteria, an antimicrobial provides selective pressures

that favour overgrowth of bacteria carrying a gene that confers resistance. The continuous use of antimicrobial agents encourages the multiplication and spread of resistant strains.

The result is that drugs which cost tens of millions of dollars to produce, and take perhaps 10 years to reach the market, are only effective for a limited time period. Examples of diseases whose agents have demonstrated drug resistance include tuberculosis, malaria, gonorrhoea and typhoid fever.

In the case of tuberculosis, poor prescribing practices or poor patient

compliance with treatment have led to the development of strains of *Mycobacterium tuberculosis* which are resistant to the available drugs. Malaria presents a double resistance problem: resistance of the *Plasmodium* parasites, which cause the disease, to antimalarial drugs; and resistance of the *Anopheles* mosquitoes, the vectors of the disease, to insecticides. Pneumococci and *Haemophilus influenzae*, the most common bacteria causing acute respiratory infections in children, are becoming more resistant to drugs. More than 90% of *Staphylococcus aureus* strains and about 40% of pneumococci strains are resistant to penicillin.

In the USA, antibiotic-resistant bacteria generate costs of a minimum of $4 billion to $5 billion yearly; these costs are likely to be much higher in developing countries.

Answering questions concerning the use of antibiotics in food production, emphasizing ways to prolong the effectiveness of existing antibiotics, pursuing key areas of basic research and seeking incentives for developing new antibiotics, and exploring legal and regulatory mechanisms in key areas of need are priorities that need to be addressed by policy-makers.

Source: **Harrison PF, Lederberg J** (eds). *Antimicrobial resistance: Issues and options.* Institute of Medicine. Washington DC, National Academy Press, 1998.

result from their *joining the curve*. That the infant mortality rate in low and middle income countries is higher in the most populous countries suggests the importance of focused international assistance. Health systems need to provide the existing, cost-effective interventions to these populations so that the countries that are currently lagging behind can join the curve.

Immunization is the greatest public health success story in history *(12)*. The basic vaccines are available to combat the six major diseases in children (measles, tetanus, pertussis, tuberculosis, poliomyelitis and diphtheria). Immunization coverage falls far short of 100%, and it is the world's poorest and most vulnerable children who remain unreached.

Poliomyelitis is an example of a disease for which eradication is possible. The only reason for the existence of remaining cases is insufficient coverage. WHO is committed to

Figure 2.6 Infant mortality rate related to income

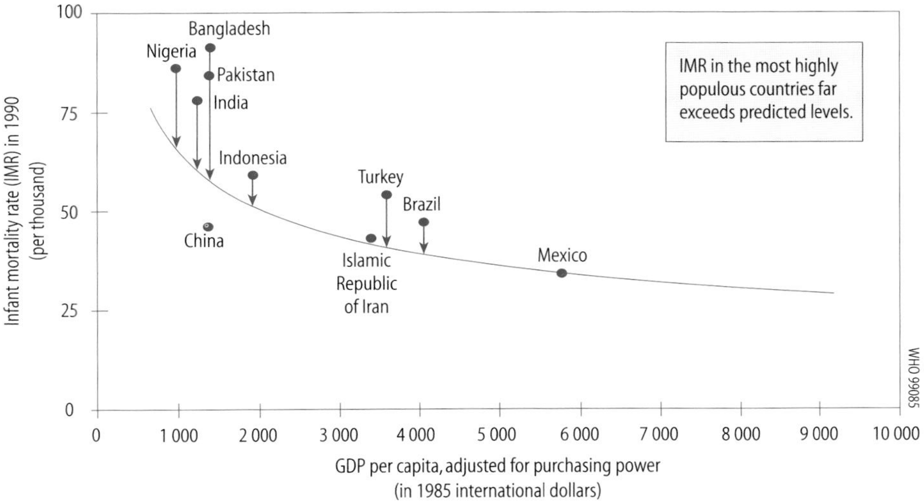

Note: For explanation of the curve ralating IMR to income, see note to Figure 1.4.

Box 2.5 Tuberculosis in the Western Pacific

The notified cases of tuberculosis in the Western Pacific Region in 1996 represented 25% of the global total, mainly because expansion of the WHO tuberculosis control strategy, particularly in China, improved case management and brought many more cases under treatment. There were 2.16 million estimated new cases in 1997, and the average case fatality rate was 20%. Coinfection with HIV is still low in the Region as a whole, but those who are coinfected with tuberculosis and HIV may reach 26 per 100 000 population by 2000. WHO has been collaborating closely in the establishment of surveillance of HIV infection among tuberculosis patients in Cambodia, Malaysia, and Viet Nam.

Data from 21 countries and areas in the Region show that the majority of cases occurred during the productive years of life. Delayed diagnosis or partial treatment often lead to longstanding lung disability and job loss, causing socioeconomic hardship. Untreated or inadequately treated tuberculosis patients spread the infection to others, especially in crowded and poor communities. Children aged 5–9 years living in urban slums in the Philippines showed more than twice the prevalence rate of infection for the general urban population: 39% of them were infected with the disease.

Tuberculosis ignores national boundaries. In Australia, Hong Kong (China), Malaysia and Singapore, the numbers of tuberculosis cases have not decreased for several years because of the increased or continued detection of new tuberculosis patients among immigrants.

The directly observed treatment, short course (DOTS) strategy was introduced in the Western Pacific in the early 1990s and is now used in 28 countries and areas; 35% of tuberculosis cases are treated with DOTS, and 55% of the total population have access to the strategy. In China, a DOTS programme supported by the World Bank is being implemented with WHO collaboration in 13 provinces. The programme has so far achieved a cure rate of over 90% and is accessible to 560 million people. In Cambodia, more than 90% of district health facilities are using DOTS as a routine strategy. In the Philippines, a new approach using DOTS began in three provinces in 1996, in collaboration with WHO, raising the cure rate from 60% to 80%. DOTS will be accessible to more than half of the total population in the country by the end of 1999.

Contributed by the WHO Regional Office for the Western Pacific.

eliminating poliomyelitis cases by the year 2000. As is shown in Figure 2.7, there have been remarkable reductions in the geographical spread of the disease since 1988. The last case caused by wild poliovirus in the Western hemisphere occurred in Junin, Peru, on 23 August 1991. The last case in WHO's Western Pacific Region was recorded in March 1997 near Phnom Penh in Cambodia. WHO has just initiated a "final stretch" effort with the goal of stopping transmission globally by December 2000, of certifying this achievement by 2005 and of stopping immunization by 2010. The eradication effort illustrates two important points. First, partnerships with nongovernmental organizations can be very productive: Rotary International has made major commitments to polio eradication and its influence with local leaders plus financial contributions (about US$ 500 million) have been critical to success. Second, properly designed, highly goal-oriented programmes can contribute importantly to health systems development.

WHO is also involved with the provision of interventions against several other infectious diseases. The Integrated Management of Childhood Illness is a group of preventive and curative interventions. The strategy focuses on pneumonia, diarrhoea, measles, malaria and malnutrition, as these account for 70% of all childhood deaths globally, but it also addresses other serious infections (for example, meningitis), other causes of febrile disease (for example, dengue) and other associated problems (such as eye problems associated with measles or vitamin A deficiency, and ear infections). Preventive interventions including immunization, support for breastfeeding and other nutrition counselling are also emphasized.

Other similar initiatives are in different stages of development and implementation. For tuberculosis, the "directly observed treatment, short course" (DOTS) intervention has been

Figure 2.7 Reductions in wild poliovirus transmission between 1988 and 1998

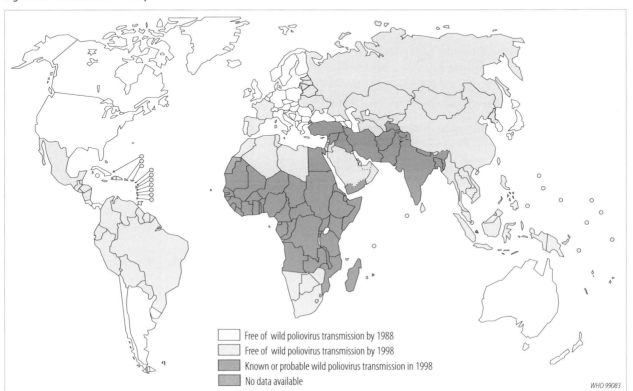

Free of wild poliovirus transmission by 1988
Free of wild poliovirus transmission by 1998
Known or probable wild poliovirus transmission in 1998
No data available

WHO 99083

shown to be highly cost-effective (see Box 2.6). Tuberculosis is highly concentrated in poor subgroups of populations, as indicated in Table 2.1. Prevalence of tuberculosis is estimated to be almost four times higher in populations living below the poverty line than in the better-off. The adult lung health initiative has grown out of the tuberculosis control activities of WHO, recognizing that only a small proportion of adults presenting with a cough have tuberculosis and that adequate treatment or advice should be provided to individuals with other lung diseases. The initiative offers an integrated approach to detecting and treating tuberculosis, asthma and chronic obstructive lung disease.

Maternal mortality risks, which are highly concentrated in developing countries, are also to a large extent preventable and avoidable. The mother–baby package aims to reduce mortality and disability associated with maternal reproductive health, the risks of delivery for both mother and child, and the first weeks of life.

At the end of the 20th century, it is unacceptable that women continue to suffer and die as a result of complications related to pregnancy and childbirth. The enormous disparities in levels of maternal mortality and morbidity between rich and poor are a continuing affront. The evidence of what works to reduce maternal mortality already exists. The interventions needed are cost-effective. Expanding health system coverage is required: women must have access to skilled assistance during pregnancy and childbirth, and they must be able to reach a functioning health care facility when complications arise.

Box 2.6 Tuberculosis and the "Stop TB" Initiative

Tuberculosis was one of the chief causes of death in northern Europe and the Americas until about 1900. Mortality rates gradually fell because of improved living conditions and the advent of effective chemotherapy, but the disease persisted in developing countries, where it causes some 25% of preventable mortality among young people. It is still a leading killer of young women worldwide. About 1.8 billion people are infected with the tuberculosis bacillus, and the tuberculosis burden will grow with an expanding global population. Inappropriate or inadequate tuberculosis treatment further increases transmission. So do such assaults on the health of the poor as hunger, civil disturbances and, most importantly, HIV which alone will account for some 14% of global cases by the year 2000.

Because tuberculosis predominantly hits young adults, its social and economic consequences are among the greatest of any infectious disease. Almost all cases are in countries least able financially to mount an effective response. In countries where resources are generally sufficient, their poor allocation and ineffective use often result in treatment which fails to cure almost all patients. These conditions explain the evolution of multidrug-resistant strains of tuberculosis.

Since 1989, WHO has encapsulated current best practice for tuberculosis case-finding and treatment into the DOTS (directly observed treatment, short course) strategy and, together with the World Bank and Harvard University, has shown it to be one of the most cost-effective health interventions available. Over 100 countries now accept DOTS as a standard approach, and over 1 million patients have been treated with it since 1990. Global surveillance systems have been established and the spread of drug resistance is being charted.

But progress is too slow, mainly because of the lack of political will and commitment within a number of high prevalence countries to broaden the deployment of the strategy to all who need it. The "Stop TB" initiative arose from discussion of these constraints between representatives of several of the high burden countries which account for 80% of the global epidemic, the International Union against Tuberculosis and Lung Disease, the Royal Netherlands Tuberculosis Association, the American Lung Association, the American Thoracic Society, the US Centers for Disease Control and Prevention, the World Bank and WHO. WHO aims to expand significantly this global coalition and to increase investment in tuberculosis control, in order to attain the Stop TB goal of reducing the tuberculosis disease burden.

The Stop TB initiative will focus on four products to accomplish its objectives.

- A global action plan to guide and accelerate coordinated responses to tuberculosis control internationally, regionally and nationally. It will offer an analytical framework and recommendations for immediate action in high burden countries and particular settings, such as areas significantly affected by multidrug-resistant strains of tuberculosis.
- A global tuberculosis drug facility to provide universal access to high quality Fixed Dose Combination preparations of anti-tuberculosis drugs and to ensure coordinated international arrangements for their financing, procurement and supply, quality control and distribution.
- A global research agenda to address short-term operational constraints and the development of new diagnostic agents, drugs and vaccines. It will facilitate collaboration on research capacity strengthening in low income, high prevalence countries; expansion of appropriate policy-relevant health systems research; control and treatment of multidrug-resistant tuberculosis; and the development of new tools.
- A global charter for advocacy and commitment to enable endemic countries and their partners to declare renewed commitment and agreement on specific steps to be taken. It will generate increased international attention to tuberculosis. Specific performance targets will enable the monitoring and reporting of progress.

Syndromic treatment of sexually transmitted infections is another example of defining best practices in the face of resource constraints. Box 2.7 describes successful interventions to stop HIV transmission in Thailand and elsewhere in South-East Asia.

Rationalization of drug use and development of drug supply systems can similarly be aided by clearly defined standard guidelines where first and second line drugs for each level are specified. Revision of the regulations on who can use which drugs is often needed. For example, an injection of quinine for severe malaria or chloramphenicol for severe pneumonia, prior to referral to a higher level in the health system, may be life saving. But health staff at first-level facilities may not be authorized to use injectable drugs or the drugs may be supplied regularly only to hospitals. Policies may need to be changed to accommodate broader use of certain drugs for defined purposes.

In addition to the disease-specific interventions and control programmes which are available, there is also a need to deal with a significant risk factor for disease, malnutrition, which is primarily concentrated in the world's poorest and most disadvantaged populations. Malnutrition is estimated to be the single most important risk factor for disease, being responsible for 16% of the global burden in 1995, measured in DALYs *(1)*. Malnutrition, either in the form of protein-energy malnutrition or micronutrient malnutrition, primarily of iron, vitamin A and iodine, often contributes to premature death, poor health, blindness, growth stunting, mental retardation, learning disabilities and low work capacity *(13,14)*. Protein-energy malnutrition, as indicated by slow or incomplete physical growth is, however, as much a consequence of disease as a cause. Infection may, in many environments, contribute more to malnutrition than dietary inadequacy. Hence disease control is important for reducing the malnutrition burden.

Box 2.7 HIV/AIDS control in South-East Asia: the challenge of expanding successful programmes

The human immunodeficiency virus (HIV) was slower to emerge in South-East Asia than in other parts of the world, but it is now a serious public health problem and a threat to development. The first patient with AIDS was reported in 1984 from Thailand, since when a total of 92 391 cases of the disease have been reported up to 1 July 1997, mostly from Thailand, India and Myanmar. However, because of under-reporting and under-diagnosis the reported cases only reflect a proportion of the true problem. UNAIDS and WHO estimate that there are currently more than 5.5 million people in WHO's South-East Asia Region (which includes India) who are infected with HIV – 18% of the global total. In 1998 alone there were estimated to be 1.2 million new infections in the Region. Heterosexual transmission may spread the virus from high-risk groups to the general population.

National authorities in the Region are responding to the pandemic with urgency. They have developed strategic plans and are implementing a variety of control measures, as the following examples show.

• Thailand's 100% condom use programme has received worldwide attention. Its effectiveness can be assessed by the declining HIV incidence among military recruits: from 3.6% in 1993 to 2.1% in 1995. At the same time, sexually transmitted diseases are at a lower rate than ever before.
• In Calcutta, India, the Sonagachi health care and education project among sex workers has become a model for successful peer education; HIV prevalence remains low and sexually transmitted diseases are declining.

• Needle exchange programmes and community-based treatment approaches for injecting drug users in Myanmar and Nepal have been effective in bringing about behavioural change and reducing HIV infection rates.

WHO continues to provide technical, material and logistical support to national programmes for AIDS prevention and the control of sexually transmitted diseases, through the Regional Office in New Delhi and in selected countries. WHO collaborates with the World Bank and with UNAIDS – of which it is a cosponsor – in assisting national programmes and in carrying out intercountry and regional activities.

The integration of care of sexually transmitted diseases into the general health services is considered a priority in the region, necessitating the train-

ing of primary care workers, managers and private practitioners. WHO and UNAIDS provide support to governments in order to monitor the trends of the HIV/AIDS pandemic through surveillance, to promote research, to ensure safe blood transfusions, and to strengthen laboratory diagnostic services. Other priority interventions include case management capacity building, health promotion and education, and the planning of comprehensive care and counselling for people with AIDS or infected with HIV.

Evidence shows that intervention can succeed. Augmented political, financial and technical support is required to make sure that interventions are delivered where they are needed.

Contributed by the WHO Regional Office for South-East Asia.

Interventions to reduce micronutrient malnutrition are likely to prove particularly cost-effective. Programmes can include four strategies – supplementation, fortification, food-based approaches leading to dietary diversification, and complementary public health control measures – to the degree appropriate and feasible *(13)*. The long-term goal of intervention should be to shift emphasis away from supplementation towards a combination of food fortification – universal salt iodization or iron-fortified flour, for example – and dietary diversification.

In conclusion, the double burden of disease defines the complexity of the problems health systems must address. The two elements of the double burden differ markedly in their implications for policy. The unfinished agenda deals with a limited number of conditions, highly concentrated on the poor and for most of which extremely cost-effective interventions are available. This burden on the poor is, indeed, an unnecessary one that targeted programmes can alleviate. Epidemiological transition, on the other hand, generates epidemiological diversity. This aspect of the double burden involves large numbers of conditions potentially affecting everyone, although here again the poor suffer more. Interventions – whether preventive or curative – are less likely to be decisive, although there are important exceptions, such as tobacco control discussed in Chapter 5. Health systems must be able to respond flexibly to this diversity.

REFERENCES

1. **Murray CJL, Lopez AD** (eds). *The global burden of disease: A comprehensive assessment of mortality and disability from diseases, injuries, and risk factors in 1990 and projected to 2020.* Cambridge, Harvard School of Public Health on behalf of the World Health Organization and The World Bank, 1996 (Global Burden of Disease and Injury Series, Vol.I).

2. **Preston SH, Keyfitz N, Schoen R**. *Causes of death: Life tables for national populations.* New York and London, Seminar Press, 1972.

3. **Frenk J et al**. Health transition in middle-income countries: new challenges for health care. *Health policy and planning,* 1989, **4**(1): 29–39.

4. *The world health report 1996 – Fighting disease, fostering development.* Geneva, World Health Organization, 1996.

5. *The world health report 1998 – Life in the 21st century: A vision for all.* Geneva, World Health Organization, 1998.

6. *World development report 1993 – Investing in health.* New York, Oxford University Press for The World Bank, 1993.

7. Editorial. The hidden epidemic of cardiovascular disease. *The Lancet,* 1998, **352**(9143):1795.

8. **Howson CP, Reddy KS, Ryan TJ, Bale JR** (eds). *Control of cardiovascular diseases in developing countries. Research, development and institutional strengthening.* Institute of Medicine. Washington DC, National Academy Press, 1998.

9. *Investing in health research and development. Report of the Ad Hoc Committee on Health Research Relating to Future Intervention Options.* Geneva, World Health Organization, 1996 (document WHO/TDR/Gen/96.1).

10. *Health situation in the Americas: Basic indicators 1998.* Washington, PAHO/WHO, 1998 (document PAHO/HDP/HDA/98.01).

11. **Harrison PF, Lederberg J** (eds). *Antimicrobial resistance: Issues and options.* Institute of Medicine. Washington DC, National Academy Press, 1998.

12. **Henderson RH**. Immunization: going the extra mile. In: *The progress of nations 1998.* New York, UNICEF, 1998.

13. **Howson CP, Kennedy ET, Horwitz A** (eds). *Prevention of micronutrient deficiencies: Tools for policymakers and public health workers.* Institute of Medicine. Washington DC, National Academy Press, 1998.

14. *WHO global database on child growth and malnutrition.* Geneva, World Health Organization, 1997 (document WHO/NUT/97.4).

PART TWO

MAKING A DIFFERENCE IN THE 21ST CENTURY

Part Two deals with three specific approaches to making a difference for better health in the 21st century. Chapter 3 poses a major question confronting health policy-makers. Can they learn from the experiences of others, or in a systematic way from their own past, about what is likely to work – and what is likely to fail – in designing health reforms? Recent experiences suggest that the answer is yes. Chapter 3 draws selected experiences together in advocating a "new universalism" as a framework for guiding health system development to meet the challenges of the 21st century.

Chapters 4 and 5 deal with major conditions representing each element of the double burden of disease described in Chapter 2. Chapter 4 focuses on malaria, a major component of the unfinished agenda of diseases of the poor. To make a difference to malaria in the 21st century, the resources of industry, government, science, and ordinary people need to be engaged. WHO's Roll Back Malaria project will combine leadership with knowledge, experience and resources to achieve major reductions in malaria morbidity and mortality in the early years of the next century.

Chapter 5 addresses tobacco, a risk factor accelerating the epidemic of noncommunicable diseases. Tobacco use will have become the biggest single cause of death by the time we enter the next century. Effective control strategies exist. Chapter 5 reviews those strategies and describes WHO's Tobacco Free Initiative, which provides a source of legal, political and financial assistance for countries and organizations fighting to control the tobacco epidemic. As a central element of its work, the initiative will generate a knowledge base of national experiences and global data for all to use.

WHO itself is changing, to focus better on the challenges of the next century. Chapter 6 summarizes the challenges and identifies areas of focus where WHO's limited resources can make the greatest difference.

3

MEETING THE CHALLENGES:
HEALTH SYSTEMS DEVELOPMENT

*I*n the early 1990s the world devoted about 9% of its total product to the health sector *(1)*. This massive commitment of resources responds to the diversity of health challenges resulting from the demographic and epidemiological transition. Chapter 2 delineated the potential that health systems now have for markedly reducing the huge amount of excess disease that the poor and disadvantaged suffer. This burden is concentrated in a very limited number of conditions, and Chapter 2 indicated how health systems could – and should – address those conditions, for which effective tools already exist. In sharp contrast to the focus that health systems can bring to the particular problems of the poor they must also anticipate and respond to a bewildering variety of diseases and injuries. The tenth revision of the International Classification of Diseases runs to over two thousand pages *(2)*. Although some of these conditions occur more frequently than others, health systems must have the financial means, organizational structures and procedures to respond flexibly and efficiently to this diversity.

The development of science-based, organized health systems is relatively recent, and very much in progress. Box 3.1 highlights some 20th century milestones in the development of health systems. Most countries have no single health system, but several distinct health financing and provision sub-systems, embracing different types of traditional or alternative practice, as well as public, private and not-for-profit hospitals and clinics, sometimes offering services for limited population sub-groups, such as civil servants.

Health systems in some countries perform well. Others perform poorly. An accumulation of applied research efforts and practical experience now suggests some reasons for these differences. Countries differ, of course, and lessons that are useful to one country may have little value to others. Furthermore, evidence about what has worked – and what has not – constitutes only one of several factors influencing the decisions that shape health systems. That said, for many government officials, as for many clinicians, evidence *does* matter. But clearly, for national purposes, only national officials can judge the relevance and political feasibility of using evidence generated from other countries and other times.

This chapter attempts, very briefly, to summarize evidence being accumulated concerning a few key questions on health system finance and development. A more detailed analysis and comparison of health system performance and policies will be the subject of *The world health report 2000*. In the meantime, WHO is being strengthened in several ways to ensure that the Organization's support for health systems development is effective. A new Global Programme on Evidence for Health Policy has been established to improve and expand the knowledge base in key areas of epidemiology and disease burden measurement, assessment of service quality and cost-effectiveness, and comparative analysis of financing, organizational, regulatory and legislative options. A regrouping of programmes in headquarters in the cluster on Health Systems and Community Health ensures that priority interventions, such as the Integrated Management of Childhood Illness (IMCI), and health systems strengthening work together in WHO's technical support to countries.

Priorities such as Roll Back Malaria and the Tobacco Free Initiative are strongly oriented to health systems strengthening. And a time-limited Cabinet project, entitled Partnerships for Health Sector Development, has been created to change the way that WHO works on health sector-wide development with national and international development agencies, within and beyond the United Nations system.

Before turning to the evidence, it is worth listing the goals of health systems – as WHO sees them. Goals can be phrased in many ways, and each goal may have different relevance in different contexts. Yet the following core list of goals for health system development is likely to elicit broad agreement:

- improving health status;
- reducing health inequalities;
- enhancing responsiveness to legitimate expectations;
- increasing efficiency;
- protecting individuals, families and communities from financial loss;

Box 3.1 Reports that have changed health systems

The three reports described below, although directed to national policy-makers, have had a profound influence on health systems throughout the world. The Alma-Ata Declaration, however, provided the first international model of a health system that would assure universal access.

The background to the **Flexner Report** (USA, 1910) was growing concern at proliferating, low-standard medical training programmes in North America. Based on a detailed assessment of medical schools in each state of the USA and province of Canada, Flexner examined the physical facilities and equipment, curriculum, financial situation, faculty qualifications and admission requirements of the great majority of medical schools. Only a tiny minority of institutions were found to be teaching a scientifically based curriculum in facilities with a hospital connection, appropriate conditions

and equipment, to men and women with an adequate educational background. His report was influential in the establishment of national admission standards requiring four years of post-secondary education, and the adoption of a four-year, science-based curriculum.

The **Dawson Report** (UK, 1920) designed a system of district health services based on general practitioners and health centres, with referral for difficult cases through first and second level health centres to teaching hospitals. Dawson's vision was to take the entire population of an area as the basis for planning: the system he proposed was a marked improvement over the haphazard mixture of personal medical care and institutional care for the sick, homeless, handicapped and poor, which characterized Britain at the beginning of the 20th century. Although Dawson's recommendations were not directly implemented on any scale, his thinking

influenced the development of local health systems for the remainder of the century.

The **Beveridge Report** (UK, 1942) provided the rationale and blueprint for Britain's post-war welfare state, weaving the separate fragments of public and charitable welfare programmes into a modern, universal system of social protection, based on a pooling of risk among the entire population. Beveridge outlined how the fragmentary and often archaic British system of charitable and public welfare benefits could be pulled together to allow the country to tackle "Want, Disease, Ignorance, Squalor and Idleness, the five giant evils on the road to reconstruction". Although health was only one area of Beveridge's concern, and the report made no detailed recommendations about how a national health service should be run, it nevertheless laid the foundations of the British National Health Service, which came into being in 1948. Both

Beveridge's ideas about compulsory social insurance and the subsequent (tax-funded) National Health Service have influenced other countries' health and social welfare systems.

The **Alma-Ata Declaration** (1978) emerged from the International Conference on Primary Health Care. Motivated by gross inequality in health status within and between countries, and arguing that health is essential to social and economic development, the Declaration identifies primary health care as the key to the attainment by the year 2000, by all people, of a level of health that will permit them to lead a socially and economically productive life. The Declaration identifies the essential elements and intersectoral nature of primary health care. All WHO Member States became signatories. Alma-Ata gave global impetus to the insight and vision of the three previous reports.

Sources:
Flexner A. *Medical education in the United States and Canada. A report to the Carnegie Foundation for the Advancement of Teaching.* New York, Carnegie Foundation, 1910.
Interim report on the future provision of medical and allied services. Report of the Dawson Committee. London, His Majesty's Stationery Office, 1920.
Social insurance and allied services. Report by Sir William Beveridge. London, His Majesty's Stationery Office, 1942.
Primary health care. Report of the International Conference on Primary Health Care, Alma-Ata, USSR, 6–12 September 1978. Geneva, World Health Organization, 1978 ("Health for All" Series, No.1).

- enhancing fairness in the financing and delivery of health care.

This chapter also considers the following questions. How can the limits to government involvement and government finance be recognized, and how can choices be made that best achieve the right balance between systemic goals while recognizing budgetary and other limits? What incentives for providers of care will constrain cost escalation while motivating compassionate service of high quality? Independently of sources of finance, what are reasonable roles for private and public providers of care to play? How can research and development to underpin continued health improvement globally be sustained in a context where most health finance is national? Finally, and most important, what is the role of government in financing health services? Analytic and empirical work provides no specific answers to these questions but, rather, assembles the evidence on consequences resulting from the choices made in different countries at different times. The accumulated evidence may, in some cases, suggest that certain policies have worked well, while others have worked poorly.

Where, to anticipate the findings of the chapter, do the values of WHO lead when combined with the available evidence? *They lead away from a form of universalism that has governments attempting to provide and finance everything for everybody.* This "classical" universalism, although seldom advanced in extreme form, shaped the formation of many European health systems. It achieved important successes. But classical universalism fails to recognize both resource limits and the limits of government.

The findings also lead away from market-oriented approaches that ration health services according to the ability to pay. Not only do market-oriented approaches to finance lead to intolerable inequity with respect to a fundamental human right, but growing bodies of theory and evidence indicate them to be inefficient as well. Market mechanisms have enormous utility in many sectors and have underpinned rapid economic growth for over a century in Europe and elsewhere. But the very countries that have relied heavily on market mechanisms to achieve the high incomes they enjoy today are the same countries that rely most heavily on governments to finance their health services. Therein lies a lesson. Health is an important component of national welfare. Achieving high health outcomes requires a combination of universal entitlement and tight control over expenditure.

This report advocates a "new universalism" that recognizes governments' limits but retains government responsibility for the leadership and finance of health systems. The new universalism welcomes diversity and, subject to appropriate guidelines, competition in the provision of services. At the same time it recognizes that if services are to be provided for all then not all services can be provided. The most cost-effective services in a given setting should be provided first. The new universalism recognizes private providers as an important source of care in many countries; welcomes private sector involvement in supplying service providers with drugs and equipment; and it encourages increased public and private investment in generating the new drugs, equipment and vaccines that will underpin long-term improvements in health.

ACHIEVING GREATER EFFICIENCY

Efficiency concepts in health systems apply at several different levels. "Macroeconomic efficiency" *(3)* refers to the total costs of health care in relation to aggregate measures of health status. Countries spend very different amounts of national resources on health, allocate those resources in very different ways, and achieve very different health outcomes in terms of health status, access or satisfaction. Some of those outcome differences point to differences in health system efficiency. China's performance (relative to national income) in reducing infant mortality fell sharply between the late 1970s and 1992, when incomes were rising but the rural medical system was deteriorating. Figure 3.1 illustrates this trend with data drawn from Annex Table 5. Comparative work in Latin America suggests that a given level of health expenditure contributes positively to reductions in under-5 mortality if it is from public sources, negatively if from private *(4)*.

Some governments have traditionally regarded health spending by the public sector as a pure consumption expenditure, and have wanted to minimize it. This is often the perspective of ministries of finance. Yet in many poor countries total health spending from all sources is very low – less than 2% of GDP in Cameroon, Indonesia, Nigeria, Sri Lanka and Sudan, for example – meaning that even the most inexpensive and effective health measures cannot be made available to the whole population. Even in Zambia, where over 3% of GDP is allocated to health, the public per capita spending (government and external assistance) is only about half of the $12 suggested by the World Bank as necessary to fund the cost of a basic package of preventive and curative interventions. The reality is that allocating an inadequate share of resources to health, from both public and private sources, perpetuates the cycle of poverty. Increased public financial support for cost-effective and equitable health services is overdue in many countries.

In middle and upper income countries, health financing policy is frequently driven by the need to increase coordination, reduce fragmentation and exert better control over total health care costs. Countries in this group are often worried that their level of health spending will threaten economic growth and competitiveness by making their labour force, and therefore goods and services, more expensive. Argentina, France, Germany, Switzerland and the USA, for example, are all spending in excess of 9% of GDP on health, and in the USA the figure has risen to 14%. While spending much more than 9% of GDP may indicate macroeconomic inefficiency, countries spending less than 2% are almost certainly investing too little in the health of their present and future population. Within this broad range there is no single economically efficient or "correct" level of funding.

"Microeconomic efficiency" refers to the scope for achieving greater efficiency from existing patterns of resource use. Wastage and inefficiency occur in all health systems. Allocative inefficiency occurs when resources are devoted to the wrong activities. Spending large amounts of the health budget on hospital-based care for children with measles is clearly an allocative inefficiency: those children should have been immunized. Well-prioritized and universally accessible service packages, of the sort discussed in Chapter 2, can make major gains in the allocative efficiency of health systems of both rich and poor countries.

Technical inefficiency occurs when too many resources are used to achieve a given health intervention or outcome. An imbalance between the installed capacity of a health system (its buildings, equipment and staff) and the recurrent resources needed for its proper functioning gives rise to a set of technical inefficiencies – with overstaffing and underemployment in relation to utilization levels becoming common, particularly at peripheral health facilities. Cost-effectiveness analysis is the key tool for guiding improvements in microeconomic efficiency.

Service quality falls when the required inputs (physical and human) are lacking, and when proper procedures are

Figure 3.1 Infant mortality rate relative to income, China, 1962–1992

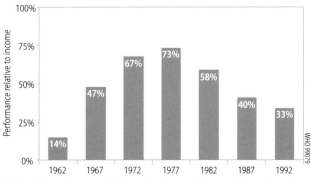

Relative performance is measured as distance from the average infant mortality rate of countries at the same level of income.
Source: Annex Table 6.

not used. Common symptoms in the public sector are a lack of essential drugs, inaccessible health facilities or absent staff, non-functioning vehicles and equipment, and dilapidated premises. Where these symptoms occur, health outcomes suffer. People's perceptions of the fairness and responsiveness of government also suffer. Comparable difficulties abound in the private sector. In the large and inadequately regulated private sector of low and middle income countries, health workers are often unqualified and diagnostic and prescribing practices are poor or even hazardous. Private sector treatment of tuberculosis, for example, often involves profitable but useless intervention while failing to achieve the high cure rates that have been attained in public facilities.

SETTING PRIORITIES

Even the wealthiest countries may not be able to provide entire populations with every intervention that has medical value. Priorities have to be debated, agreed and implemented, if universal access to affordable and effective health care is to be achieved. In most countries today, priorities are set in ways which exclude large numbers of people from access to organized care. Ability to pay appears increasingly to be the mechanism rationing access to care (5). WHO can make a major difference in helping governments to do better than this. An open and vigorous debate about how to set priorities in health has begun. Choosing public priorities, in terms of what governments will do and will not do, is how economic reality becomes an integral part of health system development and reform.

Explicit priority setting in health has taken several steps forward since the mid-1980s. National or regional guidelines have been debated, published and – to differing degrees – implemented in the Netherlands, New Zealand, Norway, Sweden and in Oregon, USA (6). Approaches differ. In Sweden, an explicit value base was proposed, of three principles in descending order of importance: human dignity regardless of personal characteristics and social functions; need and solidarity; and cost-effectiveness. Several categories of political and clinical priority were defined. In Oregon and the Netherlands, the value bases for priority setting were also explicit. They all differed.

In developing countries, the debate on priorities has often been led by international agencies. From the early 1950s to the 1980s, global public health initiatives tended to focus on a single disease at a time, such as malaria or diarrhoeal disease, and sometimes on a single intervention, such as DDT spraying or oral rehydration therapy. More recently, international advice has favoured grouped interventions, to achieve better outcomes and improve service quality. The Expanded Programme on Immunization groups vaccines aimed at preventing diphtheria, tetanus, pertussis, poliomyelitis, tuberculosis and measles.

The *World development report 1993 (7)* pushed forward debate on priority setting by introducing the notion of cost-effective intervention packages, tailored according to the public finance reality of each country. Numerous countries have designed such priority packages (8). Bangladesh, Colombia, Mexico and Zambia have begun implementation.

The clear definition of priorities facilitates planning, training, monitoring and supervision of services in districts, provided the necessary investments are made in capacity building at this level. When packages of services for the most common conditions have been developed, health facilities can be reorganized to ensure shorter waiting times, more efficient patient flow, more standardized dispensing of drugs and better communication with users of the services. In these ways, focused intervention priorities allow limited resources to have the greatest possible impact on service quality and health outcomes.

Focused approaches can reduce much of the excess disease burden of the poor, as illustrated in Chapter 2. Cost-effectiveness summarizes in a single measure the key scientific and technical evidence on health-improving actions. But without participatory processes to engage and sustain national and local debate on health priorities, the scientific information base will remain peripheral to actual implementation of resource allocation procedures in countries. Priority-setting, the way to obtain working agreement on allocative efficiency, is here to stay.

Re-thinking incentives to providers

Two further influences on efficiency and service quality are the way in which service providers are paid, and the role of budget or fund-holding agencies with respect to service providers.

The likely incentive effects of many ways in which hospitals, clinics or individual practitioners are paid have been well studied (9–11). Prospective payment methods (e.g. budgets, capitation) transfer financial risk for delivering services from budget or fund-holding institutions (e.g. village or community prepayment schemes or commercial health insurance funds) to providers. Retrospective payment methods (e.g. fee-for-service, case-based payment) reimburse providers for services rendered. It is clear from experiences in many countries at all income levels that pure fee-for-service methods (particularly those involving "third party" payment to providers) create incentives for overspending and inappropriate care. Without controls on utilization volume or quality of service, these systems are difficult to manage in the public interest and have created incentives for extravagant and wasteful care, through oversupply of medication, over-use of diagnostic services and excessive surgical intervention (12–14). Fee-for-service systems often create the wrong incentives for providers from a public policy perspective, and rapid but relatively unproductive growth in health expenditures (15). Better choices exist, ranging from sophisticated prepayment methods to fee-for-service supplemented by relatively simple administrative controls to limit cost escalation (e.g. review of prescribing patterns to ensure compliance with an essential drugs list). A major challenge for many countries is to ensure that poor quality and inefficient practice are not rewarded, whilst practice which is oriented to achieving health gain in populations is recognized in remuneration. Changing from fee-for-service to capitation in California, USA, for example, brought cost escalation there to a stop within a few years.

Prepayment means that fund-holding institutions are created: personal or family medical savings accounts, village or community schemes, private health insurance funds, health maintenance organizations, and of course public budgets for health. Many health funds have traditionally been passive financial intermediaries, failing to take full advantage of their financial power to promote changes in provider behaviour. In today's environment, however, there is a widespread tendency to explore contracting arrangements between public purchasers and different types of providers. This extends, in many countries, to relations between different parts of the public sector, for example between central and local government health bodies. Competitive pressure has had a similar effect and has driven much of the "managed care" reform in the United States; it is worth noting that much of the introduction of competition was the result of efforts by state and local government to contain cost growth in services purchased for their own employees, for the elderly or for the poor.

In the health system reforms of New Zealand and the United Kingdom, and more recently in Kyrgyzstan and Zambia, the functional distinction between funding bodies and service providers has been formalized as a "purchaser–provider split". For public hospitals, autonomy over financial and managerial decisions is being introduced or increased in many countries, with benchmarks agreed for performance monitoring. Many health insurers are taking an active role in managing the provision of care to their beneficiaries. Budget allocations to district health managers in Ghana are now managed in much the same way as contracts, with prior agreement on performance indicators and the possibility of rewards or penalties in subsequent budget allocations. These experiences reflect the same trend: a more active use of the purchasing power of fund-holding agencies to control costs and improve the quality of services provided.

Payment incentives are not the only component of a more active purchasing role by insurers or public budget-holding bodies. Other elements in active purchasing include: primary care gatekeeping to improve the efficiency of the referral process; the maintenance of provider profiles so that the purchasing agent can more actively monitor individual provider behaviour; contracting with selected providers who meet defined quality and cost criteria; utilization review and quality assurance activities to reduce inappropriate care and improve quality; and the development of standard treatment protocols, such as in prescribing or adherence to national essential drugs lists *(16)*.

Direct comparison between public and private providers of the same services, whether these are clinical or support services, opens the way for publicly managed competition between a wide array of possible providers. Competition for the delivery of health care to populations is an important means of empowering consumers vis-à-vis providers, so long as there is a well-informed and capable purchaser acting on behalf of consumers, using its financial power to induce changes in provider behaviour that improve the quality and efficiency of care for the population to which the purchaser is accountable.

Few ministries of health or public providers use mechanisms for assessing people's preferences or satisfaction with the way health services are provided. Such unresponsiveness has been part of the environment in which private provision has flourished. Private providers have often ensured that their office locations and opening times are convenient for people. Greater accountability by the public sector requires much more concern with the way people are treated by health workers, both clinically and socially.

Clear policy guidance needs to be supported by an enabling set of institutions, which offer the appropriate incentives. But there must be discretion in the interpretation of general policy guidelines to meet local circumstances and an informed, consultative and accountable chain of command, from the peripheral clinic or health post to the minister's office. Achieving such a system often requires far-reaching change from the health system models in many countries, where the public sector is typically subject to centralized control, while the private sector is virtually unsupervised.

RENEWING PROGRESS TOWARDS UNIVERSAL COVERAGE

A clear historical lesson emerges from health systems development in the 20th century: spontaneous, unmanaged growth in any country's health system cannot be relied upon to ensure that the greatest health needs are met *(17,18)*. Public intervention is necessary to achieve universal access. In any country, the greatest burden of ill-health and the biggest risk of avoidable morbidity or mortality are borne by the poor. While progress towards universal access to health care of an acceptable quality has been substantial in this century (as illustrated by global immunization coverage, see Figure 3.2), the distribution of services in most countries of the world remains highly skewed in favour of the better-off. While the equity arguments for universal public finance are widely accepted, what is less well known is that this approach achieves greater efficiency as well.

Figure 3.2 Global immunization coverage, 1987–1997

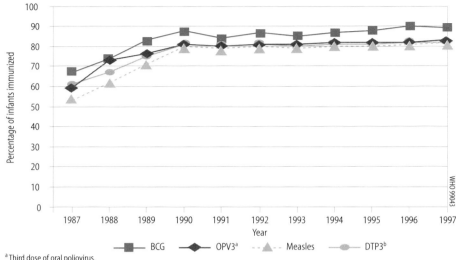

^a Third dose of oral poliovirus.
^b Third dose of diphtheria-tetanus-pertussis.

RISK SHARING

Figure 3.3 illustrates how different types of financing schemes and provider payment systems distribute the risk of health care costs differently. In the simplest payment schemes (bottom left segment), the patient pays the doctor's full costs directly, out of pocket, when he or she is ill and needs care. This is a "first party" payment system: the entire burden of risk for the financial consequences of sickness is borne by the individual and possibly by his or her family. There is little or no spreading of risks among the population. This type of arrangement probably characterizes most primary health care transactions in poor countries today, especially for care provided by so-called "traditional" practitioners.

Family, kinship-based and other forms of voluntary risk sharing (moving clockwise from the lower left) mean that risks are being shared among larger groups. Some insurance funds may pay providers directly, usually reimbursing them according to an agreed schedule of charges. The element of pre-payment is an indicator of the locus of risk shifting from the individual to the group or fund. Towards the apex of the figure are systems which pool risks among large populations – to the left of the apex are systems in which private insurers manage funds on behalf of large groups of people and reimburse providers accordingly, and to the right are general tax-funded national health systems and payroll tax-funded social health insurance systems. Most health services are paid for from one of these large funds which are "third party" payers. A wide range of options for the payment of providers exists within this spectrum of organizational arrangements. Combinations of payment methods are increasingly common. Financial risk rests with the third party (the health fund or budget-holder), though a variety of mechanisms may ensure that the patient also contributes or that some of the risk is transferred to providers, either individually or in groups.

Movement down the right segment increasingly involves the provider of care as a "second party" in sharing the risks of health care costs. When providers (hospitals or individual practitioners) manage the health needs of a population from a given budget, their own remuneration may fluctuate according to the type and level of care they provide. In this way providers become stakeholders in the active management of the health risks and needs of a population.

Figure 3.3 Who bears the risk of health care costs? The impact of different financing schemes and provider payment systems

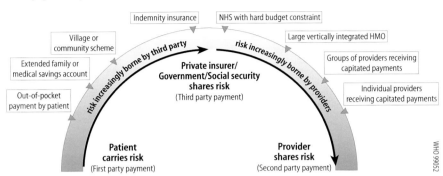

HEALTH CARE COVERAGE

The two decades since the Alma-Ata Declaration have not seen the realization of the wished-for rapid and sustained progress towards universally accessible basic health care. The global picture is very uneven, with many countries dismantling their social protection mechanisms in health rather than expanding them. Major shifts in the 1990s in formerly socialist countries towards market economies have often been accompanied by a widespread movement of the health workforce into private practice, particularly in urban areas. In the decades up to the 1980s, many socialist countries had established universally accessible health care systems. Although these may have been inefficient, bureaucratic and unresponsive to patients' needs, basic care and, in many cases, secondary and tertiary care as well, was effectively prepaid and available to almost the entire population for little or no payment at the time of need. Most people in these countries have found that they have now to pay more – officially or unofficially – for their health care, and access to care is increasingly reflecting the ability to pay. In just a decade, China dismantled its Rural Cooperative Medical System, built up from the 1950s to provide health insurance protection for the great majority, and in the 1980s made some four-fifths of the total population uninsured, in other words fully responsible for their own health care costs. Figure 3.4 summarizes this fall in coverage, and the dramatic decrease in protection of the rural population. In sub-Saharan Africa, user fees for health care have been instituted or increased in the great majority of countries *(19)*. Frequently, these policies missed opportunities to use fee revenues to improve the quality and availability of services. Attendance rates, particularly at public primary health facilities, are often already very low, indicating that most people now prefer to use traditional or private sector providers of primary care.

The industrialized countries have largely preserved their systems of near-universally accessible and prepaid health care, sometimes (as in Canada, New Zealand and the United Kingdom) implementing major organizational reform programmes. However, the fraction of the population under age 65 without private or public insurance protection in the United States has continued to grow, from nearly 15% in 1987 to nearly 18% in 1996 *(20)*. And other countries have begun to shift payment responsibilities for long term care directly onto patients and their families. Inequality in health outcomes between the poorest and best-off groups have widened in many industrialized countries. Yet some countries have made real progress towards universal coverage. The Republic of Korea implemented uni-

Figure 3.4 **Health insurance status of China's population, 1981 and 1993**

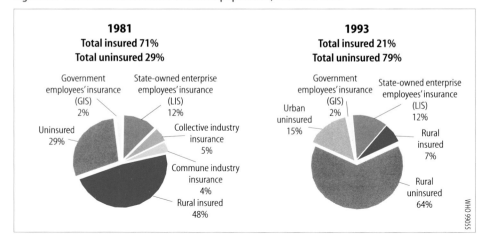

versal health insurance in 1989, during a long period of rapid economic growth. In 1993, Egypt extended health insurance protection to cover schoolchildren, increasing coverage from 4.9 million to over 20 million people. Many countries have nascent social insurance schemes.

POLICY CHOICES

Some, but by no means all, health policy choices involve trade-offs among the goals set out at the beginning of this chapter. As China's and Sri Lanka's experience in the 1950s and 1960s has shown, in situations of great poverty it is possible to make dramatic improvements in equitable access to care and simultaneously to bring about major improvements in health outcomes, while still keeping total public spending on health at modest levels.

Box 3.2 Macroeconomic and health benefits of universal mandatory health insurance: the Canadian experience

In the mid-1960s most of Canada's population had private health insurance protection provided through employers, although a substantial minority remained uninsured. This situation resembles that in the USA today. National Health Insurance (NHI) was phased in to each of Canada's provinces at different times between 1962 and 1971, thus creating a large-scale natural experiment. Recent analytical work comparing Canadian provinces with NHI to those with private insurance has allowed both the health and economic effects of the change to be identified and measured.

A substantial change in health care use occurred rapidly after the introduction of NHI, but little evidence was found of increased total consumption of health care: what happened was a redistribution of health resources towards more preventive care and better access for the poor. Implementation of NHI clearly improved infant health outcomes: infant mortality declined by 4% and the incidence of low birth weight declined by 1.3% for the total population (and by 8.9% for single parents).

NHI was financed for the most part by increased payroll taxes, which would be thought likely by many economists to reduce both employment levels and wages. However, Ca-

nadian provinces implementing NHI experienced an increase of over 2% in employment and of 3–4% in wages, with no change in the average number of hours worked. The authors of the study suggest that workforce productivity improved with NHI either because of greater job mobility or better health (and lower absenteeism), or both.

These results, though based on one country only, provide important empirical insights into contradictory predictions from economic theory. Standard theories of labour market behaviour predict that publicly financed health insurance, by increasing taxation, will drive down total employment

and wage levels. On the other hand, theoretical analyses of markets for health services and for health insurance conclude that free markets in these areas may lead to great inefficiency. The data from Canada provide clear evidence suggesting that NHI can create a "win-win" situation, where both health and the economic conditions of the labour force improve. For many low and middle income countries considering alternative policy directions, this provides evidence that efficiency considerations join equity ones in favouring mandatory universal coverage.

Sources: **Gruber J, Hanratty M**. The labor-market effects of introducing national health insurance: evidence from Canada. *Journal of business and economic statistics*, 1995, **13** (2): 163–173.
  Hanratty M. Canadian national health insurance and infant health. *American economic review*, 1996, **86** (1): 276–284.

Canada's shift to national health insurance simultaneously achieved both better health and economic gains (see Box 3.2). Ensuring that poor people benefit from the promotive, preventive and curative interventions that are already available not only improves their access to health care, it substantially contributes to reducing the total burden of illness facing a region or a country. Opportunities now exist to make huge inroads into avoidable health problems, whilst cementing solidarity between different social strata.

To achieve this potential, the poorest and sickest people have to be reached by health promotion and prevention programmes, and they have to be able to get to clinics or health posts (private, public or nongovernment) where the right kind of treatment is available for common local, treatable conditions. And there must be no significant price barrier at the time poor people need services. Universal coverage means that, irrespective of the source of funds, the health care system functions like a national health insurance system, prepaid either through tax revenues or through employment-based social insurance, to ensure the largest possible pool of risks. There has to be a shift in the mentality of the system from funding the "needs" of the service delivery infrastructure to purchasing services according to the health care needs of the population. Instead of a series of independent and uncoordinated insurance and health financing schemes, each with its own beneficiaries, benefits and sometimes with its own set of health facilities and professionals, a national health insurance system means a merging of risk protection responsibilities into the largest possible pool, or coordination of the benefit packages financed from different funding sources, with the ultimate aim of funding a comprehensive set of covered services from the resources of a single fund. A single fund for the pooling of risks allows for many options in the way incentives are set for individual providers of care, including the option of shifting risk to providers.

Figure 3.5 shows how risk pooling in health, and the share of public spending in total, increase as countries move away from out-of-pocket payment methods. Various institutional alternatives exist for achieving universal coverage. Recent comparative research, measuring equity in both the financing burden and the use of services by different income groups in countries, shows that the least organized and most inequitable way of paying for health care is on an out-of-pocket basis; people pay for their medical care when they need and use it. The financing burden falls disproportionally on the poorest (who face higher health care costs than the better-off), and the financial barrier means that use of services is lower among the lower income groups, in spite of their need being typically higher *(21)*.

The market response to a user-fee based system is through the development of private insurance. Insurers see a profitable opportunity. People prepay through insurance premiums, so that they do not have to live with unpredictably large health care bills. This method of financing entails some pooling of risks among the insured, but creates access inequities between the insured, who will get preferential access to better care, and the non-insured. Experience with commercial health insurance markets shows that they are both unstable and difficult to regulate, with each insurer constantly adjusting the risk profile of the beneficiary group in order to ensure that revenues are greater than expenditures.

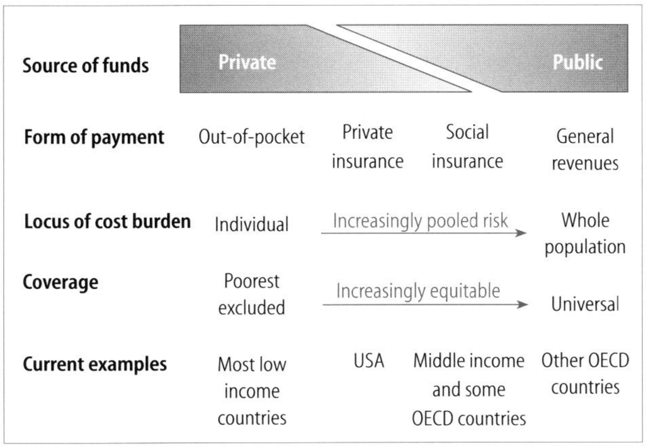

In countries with a substantial percentage of the population employed in the formal sector of the economy, a larger pooling of risks is possible through social insurance schemes,

Figure 3.5 Funding, risk pooling and coverage patterns

Source of funds	Private			Public
Form of payment	Out-of-pocket	Private insurance	Social insurance	General revenues
Locus of cost burden	Individual	Increasingly pooled risk →		Whole population
Coverage	Poorest excluded	Increasingly equitable →		Universal
Current examples	Most low income countries	USA	Middle income and some OECD countries	Other OECD countries

WHO 99054

where mainly employed people and their immediate families are compulsorily enrolled in health insurance, and where premium payments are related to each member's income, rather than their actuarial risk of illness. In Costa Rica, Germany and Japan, and in other countries where formal employment levels are high, this method of risk pooling forms the basis of the national health insurance system. In both its financing and in the access to health care that it allows, this type of system is more equitable than the two systems described above. But this conclusion does not necessarily hold true in countries where only a small percentage of the population works in the formal sector.

Most equitable of all in terms of the way the health financing burden is shared, and in allowing equal access to care for people with comparable need, are risk pooling systems based on tax revenue financing, such as in Canada, Cuba, Denmark, New Zealand, Norway, Spain, Sweden and the United Kingdom. The risk pool is the entire resident population, and the insurance function against the costs of health care is implemented by government, funded by taxes which, in a progressive system, take a larger share of income from the rich than from the poor.

Figure 3.6 shows, in simplified way, the policy options open to countries in moving towards a higher level of prepayment for health. The vertical axis represents a strategy based on the growth of private voluntary insurance schemes, in which government takes only a supportive financing role. Switzerland and the United States are illustrated as examples of this approach. The horizontal axis represents strategies in which government takes responsibility for the development of a national prepaid system based on social insurance and public finance. France and Sweden figure as examples. The shaded area close to the origin reflects existing levels of out-of-pocket payment, and the large dot close to the horizontal axis represents a low income country. What does each strategy entail for a developing country? Moving vertically is the market-oriented route, which may be preferred by better-off members of the population, but will exacerbate inequities in access. Its regulation, and overall expenditure control, will be problematic. And where formal employment levels are low as a percentage of total – as in most low and middle income countries – the level of coverage through prepayment will remain low. Only in upper middle income countries, or in situations of exceptionally high and sustained growth (over many decades in Germany and Japan, though dramatically shorter periods in the Republic of Korea and Taiwan, China), when the employment structure shifts from rural self-employment to urban formal employment, have voluntary insurance schemes grown widely enough to become the basis for a national prepaid system. The alternative strategy, along the horizontal axis, is to build prepayment systems through a combination of social insurance and public finance. Almost all countries already have elements of both, but these are seldom linked as part of an explicit health policy. Developing a national strategy for prepayment requires re-thinking public finance for health into an integrated framework of finance for universal coverage. In this, employment-based, municipal or community-based health insurance schemes would be linked with public subsidies, and guidelines given for the development of population-based coverage to ensure both equity and allocative efficiency.

Figure 3.6 Alternatives for moving towards prepaid health services

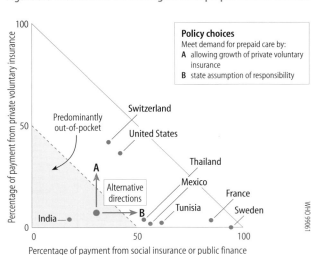

WHO 99061

New universalism

To maximize the efficiency and equity gains, and create "win-win" situations in poorer countries with large burdens of illness, practical steps towards universal coverage need to be taken. There is no single blueprint available for replication by all countries. But a number of key design features for progress to a new universalism in health are now apparent.

- *Membership is defined to include the entire population, i.e. it is compulsory.*
  Whether this is by citizenship or residence, the purpose is to ensure that the population covered is defined inclusively.

- *Universal coverage means coverage for all, not coverage of everything.*
  The prepayment system, financed by government, corporations and better-off individuals, will reflect a country's overall level of economic development. It will be a limited fund, not able to pay for all of those services that the population – and the health workforce – would like to see provided at no charge. Lower priority services, which will vary from one country to another, will only be available for payment. A benefit package has to be clearly defined in the light of the resources available and the cost of top priority health interventions, an assessment of the services and inputs for which individuals are able and willing to pay out of their own pockets, and the political feasibility of various choices.

- *Provider payment is not made by the patient at the time he or she uses the health service.*
  Health care always has to be paid for. But the way it is paid for makes a major difference to who gets care and to overall levels of health. Out-of-pocket payments penalize the cash poor: those who work outside the cash economy, or who have only seasonal or occasional cash income, or who are unemployed. Heavy reliance on out-of-pocket payment sets the wrong incentives for both users and providers, and results in an inequitable financing burden and barriers to access for the poorest. Prepayment allows a wide range of incentive-setting methods for the efficient purchasing of services.

- *Services may be offered by providers of all types.*
  Provided that health practices and health facilities meet certain quality standards and that they are subject to similar levels of managerial flexibility, their ownership status should not matter. A stronger purchaser setting standard rates of remuneration and enforcing a common set of quality and utilization regulations will enable the most efficient provider of services to flourish. Such arrangements will allow the very large numbers of private providers, who are essentially the first points of contact with the health system in many low-income countries, to be brought within a structured but pluralistic health care system, benefiting from its resources and subject to sanction and regulation by professional and public bodies.

Advice on health policy and financing from major global and regional development agencies is increasingly convergent and supportive of these messages (Box 3.3).

Providing for the Future:
the Role of Research and Development

Most discussions of health systems and health finance focus on delivering services. This is in some respects appropriate since only about 3% of health expenditures globally address the building of future capacity through research and development (R&D). Yet Chapter 1 pointed to the generation and utilization of new knowledge as the dominant force underlying the 20th century revolution in health. Health systems therefore have a responsibility to provide for the generation of new knowledge.

Health R&D entails consequences for costs of health systems as well as for outcomes. A recent review (22) identified three established directions in R&D – a revolution in biotechnology, enhanced efficiency in new pharmaceuticals development, and improved knowledge of how individuals can control their own health – that could stabilize expenditures on ageing populations. Even today's technologies, which often increase expenditure, may result in less than anticipated cost increases as populations become more elderly. This results from a steady decline in disability rates among the aged and reduced health care costs in the final years of life among the very old relative to the old. In the United States, for example, health care expenditures in the final two years before a death at age 67 exceed those before a death at age 90 by a factor of 3. These trends combine with probable cost-saving (and health-enhancing) products in today's R&D pipeline to counter demographic pressures on health expenditures. Important among these products will be improved means for health promotion and delivery of preventive care (23).

A recent WHO report (24) points to critical gaps in knowledge and needs for products, as well as to the growing productivity or capacity of the research and development enterprise itself. It presents, in short, an agenda for action that is partially at the national level

---

Box 3.3 Public finance of health systems: converging views from development agencies

Increasing agreement now replaces an early diversity of views from influential development agencies on health finance – both in terms of what should be done by governments and what should be avoided.

The importance of public finance for universal coverage was emphasized in the World Bank's *World development report 1993 – Investing in health,* with its focus on "essential services" packages. Package content would reflect each country's own preferences, but the World Bank observed that virtually all high income countries had achieved efficiency as well as equity objectives by including most services in their packages. The Inter-American Development Bank (IADB), in its 1996 report *Economic and social progress in Latin America,* likewise advocates government financing of clinical services

for reasons of efficiency as well as equity. The World Bank's 1997 Sector Strategy paper for health, nutrition and population puts the matter this way: *"The experience of most... countries suggests that governments must play a major role in health financing through regulations, mandates, and direct subsidies. Although considerable private resources may be available, these resources are often wasted on ineffective care without effective government policies."*

These agencies convey reservations, on the other hand, about the viability of private health insurance and the utility of user fees for achieving efficient and equitable health care. Contrasting the insurance experience in Chile (encouragement of private insurers) with that of Colombia (obligatory and universal membership), the IADB comments on "opportunistic behav-

iour" of private insurers, resulting in the public sector becoming increasingly responsible for the high-risk, high-cost segment of the population. The Asian Development Bank urges the gradual expansion of social health insurance and a cautious approach to cost recovery. The World Bank's 1997 paper states: "Because of the cost and the pronounced market failure that occurs in private health insurance, this is not a viable option for risk pooling at the national level in low and middle income countries." On user fees, the same paper asserts that to avoid the equity and efficiency problems associated with extensive reliance on user fees, governments must ensure that a large share of health finance derives from prepaid revenue sources.

A forum of African governments, nongovernmental organizations, bilateral and multilateral agencies recently agreed on a 15-point set of principles

on cost-sharing in education and health in sub-Saharan Africa, of which the first begins: "cost-sharing in the form of user charges should be considered only after a thorough examination of other options for financing ... other forms of government revenue are more effective, efficient and equitable."

It is important to note that these agencies' arguments for public finance rely principally on failures of private markets to deal well with problems of incomplete information, information imbalances and risk. Arguments for public finance based on "externalities" (e.g. cure of an individual tuberculosis patient reduces transmission to others) or "public goods" (e.g. a radio spot warning against smoking that can be received by all) provide a much more limited rationale for public involvement in health finance.

Sources:
World development report 1993 – Investing in health. New York, Oxford University Press, The World Bank, 1993.
Sector strategy: Health, nutrition and population. Washington DC, The World Bank, 1997.
Making social services work. Special section in: *Economic and social progress in Latin America, Report of the IADB.* Washington DC, Johns Hopkins University Press, 1996.
Policy for the health sector. Manila, Asian Development Bank, 1999.
Consensus on principles of cost-sharing in education and health in sub-Saharan Africa. Reports of an International Forum, Addis Ababa, 1997.

and partially international. The report states the case for collaboration among national health systems as follows.

"Global challenges demand, in some sense, a global response. All nations share the fruits of research and development. Even though each country may invest a relatively modest sum towards collective goals, the aggregate effort potentially benefits all substantially. Collective action is the economically rational approach to public goods such as research and development; here, responsibility for catalysing collective action lies principally in the hands of the global community. Far from overshadowing action at the national level, global efforts help both to make national research and development efforts more productive and to lead to a global result that exceeds the sum of national ones. Thus, among the many competing demands on the funds allocated to international assistance for health, those contributing to generation of the new knowledge, products and interventions that can be shared by all have special merit."

The World Bank, in two of its recent *World development reports (25,26)*, has also emphasized the importance of new knowledge for development, and that countries and the international system should collaborate in its generation.

One important step towards linking national health systems (and their research arms) into an international network has been the creation of the Global Forum for Health Research (Box 3.4). The Forum's purposes included informed advocacy for reallocation of resources towards research and development, and improving the focus and efficiency of resources now being spent. The participation of national health systems in the generation of new knowledge provides dual benefits: it quickens the overall pace of advance, and it shortens the time it takes for results to be translated into practice. Hence the importance, in planning the financing and organization of health systems, of ensuring an adequate research and development base.

Box 3.4 Investing in health research and development for the poor: the Global Forum for Health Research

Of the US$ 50–60 billion spent worldwide each year on health research by the private and public sectors combined, only 10% is devoted to the health problems of 90% of the world's population. The 1996 WHO report, *Investing in health research and development (24)*, recommended the creation of a Global Forum for Health Research to help to correct this so-called 10/90 gap. The Global Forum, established in 1997, aims at helping to bring together a wide range of partners, in the belief that adequate solutions to the present challenge of underinvestment in health research and development for the poor will require multiple participation.

The Global Forum is an international nongovernmental foundation hosted by WHO in Geneva. Much of its work is designed to foster greater efficiency in the use of existing research and development resources by providing analyses that help researchers, product developers and funders to focus on the highest priorities. It actively supports the following initiatives.

- The *Alliance for Health Policy and Systems Research* was created in response to concern that research in this area had been neglected in middle and low income countries.
- The *Global Tuberculosis Research Initiative* is being established to provide a coordinated response to the increasing global incidence of the disease, low uptake of the DOTS treatment strategy, increasing resistance to existing remedies, and the spread of tuberculosis related to the HIV/AIDS pandemic.
- An *Initiative for the Control of Cardiovascular Diseases (CVD)* in developing countries is being established as an outcome of recent studies, such as the World Bank-funded study by the US Institute of Medicine. This study predicts that in middle and low income countries there will be a rapid rise in the global CVD burden from 10% in 1990 to 15% in 2020. There is an urgent need to develop strategies and cost-effective interventions for dealing with this problem.
- The *Initiative on Health and Societies* plans to identify and study the key determinants of health outside the health sector, such as poverty, education, water and sanitation, and culture.
- The *Initiative on Prevention of Violence and Injuries* will contribute to a coordinated global response to the increasing problem of violence and injuries, which has hitherto been approached in a piecemeal way.
- The *Initiative on Domestic Violence against Women (including Child Abuse)* is being planned by a number of partners in response to the lack of studies on this increasing global problem. Domestic violence against women is widespread but the global disease burden is unknown.
- The *Public/Private Partnership against Malaria* aims to develop new antimalarial drugs in collaboration with the private sector.

To enable the whole population of even the richest country to have access to effective care of good quality, many choices have to be made. These choices concern health interventions, as well as the way these interventions are delivered through health systems. In both cases, choices should take account of research into effectiveness in order to ensure the development of an optimal strategy. An open and informed debate about priorities in health is also a necessary part of this strategy. Informing this debate is a critical task for research, and it is one being addressed by WHO's new Global Programme on Evidence. Unless these choices are made by responsible authorities, nationally and locally, and their implementation is monitored, service provision always tends to favour the better-off groups, both in terms of where services are available and what services are offered. The objectives enumerated at the beginning of this chapter are more likely to be achieved when appropriate political and financial mechanisms complement performance data in making authorities accountable to the populations they are meant to serve. To select key interventions and to orient health services towards entire populations combines universalism with economic realism. This "new universalism" is an attainable goal for the early years of the next century.

REFERENCES

1. *Sector strategy: Health, nutrition and population.* Washington DC, The World Bank, 1997.

2. *International statistical classification of diseases and related health problems (ICD-10), Tenth revision 1992.* Geneva, World Health Organization, 1992–1994.

3. **Hurst J.** *The reform of health care: A comparative analysis of seven OECD countries.* Paris, OECD, 1992.

4. **Jamison D et al.** Income, mortality and fertility in Latin America: Country-level performance, 1960–1990. *Revista de analisis economico,* 1996, **11**(2): 219–261.

5. **Ensor T, San PB.** Access and payment for health care: The poor of northern Vietnam. *International journal of health planning and management,* 1996, 11: 69–83.

6. **Ham C.** Priority setting in health care: Learning from international experience. *Health policy,* 1997, **42**(1): 49–66.

7. *The world development report 1993 – Investing in health.* New York, Oxford University Press for The World Bank, 1993.

8. **Bobadilla J, Cowley P.** Designing and implementing packages of essential health services. *Journal of international development,* 1995, **7**: 543–554.

9. **Saltman RB, Figueras J** (eds). *European health care reform: Analysis of current strategy.* Copenhagen, WHO Regional Office for Europe, 1997 (WHO Regional Publications, European Series No. 72).

10. **Newhouse JP.** Reimbursing health plans and health providers: Efficiency in production versus selection. *Journal of economic literature,* 1996, **34**: 1236–1263.

11. **Barnum H, Kutzin J, Saxenian H.** Incentives and provider payment methods. *International journal of health planning and management,* 1995, **10**: 23–45.

12. **Medici AC et al.** Managed care and managed competition in Latin America and the Caribbean. In: Schiefer G (ed). *Innovations in health and financing.* Washington DC, The World Bank, 1997 (World Bank discussion paper No. 365).

13. **Yang BM.** The role of health insurance in the growth of the private health sector in Korea. In: Newbrander W (ed). *Private health sector growth in Asia: Issues and implications.* Chichester, John Wiley & Sons Ltd, 1997.

14. **Hsiao WC.** The Chinese health care system: Lessons for other nations. *Social science and medicine,* 1995, **41**(8): 1047–1055.

15. **McGreevey WP.** The high costs of health care in Brazil. *Bulletin of the Pan American Health Organization,* 1988, **22**(2): 145–166.

16. **Kane N.** Costs, productivity and financial outcomes of managed care. In: Saltman R, von Otter C (eds). *Implementing planned markets in health care: Balancing social and economic responsibility.* Milton Keynes, Open University Press, 1995.

17. **Arrow KJ.** Uncertainty and the welfare economics of medical care. *American economic review,* 1963, **53**: 941–973.

18. **Barr N.** *The economics of the welfare state. Second edition.* California, Stanford University Press, 1993.

19. **Nolan B, Turbat V.** *Cost recovery in public health services in sub-Saharan Africa.* Washington DC, The World Bank, 1995 (EDI Technical Materials).

20. **Hoffman C.** *Uninsured in America: A chart book.* Washington DC, Kaiser Commission on Medicaid and the Uninsured, 1998.

21. **Doorslaer E, Wagstaff A, Rutten F.** *Equity in the finance and delivery of health care: An international perspective.* Oxford, Oxford University Press, 1993.

22. **Pardes H et al.** Effects of medical research on health care and the economy. *Science,* 1999, **283**: 36–37.

23. **Freis JF et al.** Reducing health care costs by reducing the need and demand for medical services. *New England journal of medicine,* 1993, **329**: 321–325

24. *Investing in health research and development. Report of the Ad Hoc Committee on Health Research Relating to Future Intervention Options.* Geneva, World Health Organization, 1996 (document WHO/TDR/Gen/96.1).

25. *World development report 1997 – The state in a changing world.* Washington DC, The World Bank, 1997.

26. *World development report 1998/1999 – Knowledge for development.* Washington DC, The World Bank, 1998.

4

ROLLING BACK MALARIA

*M*alaria and underdevelopment are closely intertwined. Over 40% of the world's population live where there is a risk of malaria. The disease causes widespread premature death and suffering, imposes financial hardship on poor households, and holds back economic growth and improvements in living standards. It is time for a major attack on malaria. Roll Back Malaria is a new, health sector-wide partnership to combat the disease at global, regional, country and local levels. Its strategy is outlined at the end of this chapter.

THE CHALLENGE OF MALARIA

Malaria flourishes in situations of social and environmental crisis, weak health systems and disadvantaged communities. Its ability to develop resistance makes malaria a formidable adversary. Effective interventions are available but they are not reaching the people with the greatest burden of malaria because the capacity for malaria control is inadequate in endemic countries, where health systems are often weak. Better use must be made of current knowledge, new products and state-of-the-art technologies to overcome the barrier to human progress which malaria poses.

THE HEALTH BURDEN

Almost 300 million clinical cases of malaria occur worldwide each year and over one million people die (see Annex Table 8). Almost 90% of these deaths occur in sub-Saharan Africa, where young children are the most affected. Malaria is directly responsible for one in five childhood deaths in Africa and indirectly contributes to illness and deaths from respiratory infections, diarrhoeal disease and malnutrition. Though malaria is still a big problem, huge progress has been made since the beginning of the century; its recent resurgence in Africa contrasts dramatically with the global decline in mortality since 1900 (see Box 4.1).

The rapid spread of resistance to antimalarial drugs presents a potentially devastating threat to effective treatment. Safe, effective and affordable options are quickly running out, and the discovery of new antimalarials is not keeping pace. For decades chloroquine was the main drug used, but increasing resistance forced its replacement in parts of Asia and South America during the 1980s, and in the 1990s African countries are starting to follow suit.

If malaria is diagnosed and treated promptly the infection may quickly subside, but without effective treatment, severe complications – such as cerebral malaria, severe anaemia or multiple organ failure – can rapidly develop, leading to case fatality rates of 10–30%. The progression from mild symptoms to death can be rapid. Mortality is not the only problem. With hundreds of infective bites per person/year leading to frequent illness, morbidity is high. Serious long-term neurological disabilities are experienced in 10% of children hospitalized in Kenya with severe malaria. Less obvious disabilities, including impairment of cognitive development, are probably even more common.

The scale of the problem in many countries appears to be increasing. Furthermore, the number of malaria epidemics is growing both because of climatic and environmental

Box 4.1 Malaria-related mortality in the 20th century

During the first half of the 20th century the world sustained around 2 million deaths from malaria each year, most in the Asian and the Pacific tropics, and somewhat fewer in Africa. Following the end of the Second World War, national malaria control campaigns were initiated or intensified in the most affected countries, from the Middle East, through the Indian subcontinent and South-East Asia to the islands of the Western Pacific, including those of Indonesia and the Philippines. Using DDT spraying of homes (a method intended to attack the mosquito vectors of malaria where they contact the human host), spectacular reductions in malaria incidence and malaria-related mortality were achieved, especially in India and Ceylon (now Sri Lanka). The zenith of success was reached by the mid-1960s. In subsequent decades, however, the economic and political costs of sustaining the intensive efforts involved in the initial campaigns, combined with emerging resistance of the parasites and their vectors to the chemicals used to attack them, led to the resurgence of malaria transmission throughout southern Asia and the Western Pacific. Most damaging has been the emergence of multi-drug and chloroquine resistant *Plasmodium falciparum*, which, starting in the mid-1960s, has spread outwards from a focus in South-East Asia. Notwithstanding these serious setbacks, a return to the previously high malaria-related mortality rates within this vast sec-

tion of the human population has never been remotely approached. The sustained reduction of malaria-related mortality in a region from the Mediterranean to the Western Pacific in the second half of the 20th century has been an outstanding, if precarious, success in the improvement of human health.

In China, the emergence of a strong national government shortly after the end of the Second World War, and the absence of warfare itself, must have contributed to significant reductions of the malaria burden in the decades that followed. However, political turmoil within China at first prevented major advances. Then in the mid-1970s, a determined anti-malaria campaign was initiated which integrated vector control with rigorous malaria case detection and treatment. Malaria-related deaths in China are now about one

hundred per year compared with the hundreds of thousands per year through the early decades of the century. An important outcome of the Chinese anti-malaria campaign has been the development of the artemisinin derivatives of quinhaosu, a traditional Chinese herbal medicine, to combat chloroquine-resistant *P. falciparum*. In Asia and particularly in Viet Nam in the early 1990s, the use of artemisinin derivatives has dramatically reversed the general rise in malaria mortality rates in the region.

By contrast relatively little effort has been put into trying to control the malaria situation in sub-Saharan Africa. The reasons are several. In the early part of the century, African malaria was a minor part of the global problem. This was because adults in African populations were apparently unaffected, malaria-related morbidity and

mortality being limited to young children – the effect of intense infection rates leading to death or full protective immunity by mid-childhood. At a practical level, however, the intensity of malaria transmission in sub-Saharan Africa, through hugely efficient mosquito vectors, and the poverty and size of the countries facing the problem, meant that large reductions in malaria-related mortality were thought unattainable by means largely based on vector control, which were being used successfully elsewhere.

Nevertheless, malaria-related deaths in Africa, which can never have been fewer than hundreds of thousands per year, did show evidence of per capita decline from the 1950s to the early 1980s. This can probably be attributed to slowly improving living conditions and access to cheap and effective chloroquine. However, the slow downward trend in malaria-related mortality in Africa seems to have undergone a reversal, starting from the late 1980s. In relation to total population, the numbers of childhood deaths from malaria in Africa may, at the very end of the 20th century, be substantially higher than they were 10 years previously. The factor most likely to underlie such an increase in malaria-related mortality rates is the spread of chloroquine-resistant *P. falciparum* across Africa.

Contributed by Richard Carter, University of Edinburgh, Scotland.

Malaria mortality annual rates since 1900

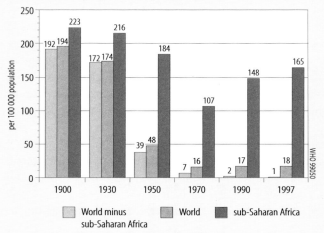

changes, and as a result of human migration, often caused by military conflicts and civil unrest.

THE ECONOMIC BURDEN

Malaria-endemic countries are some of the world's most impoverished. Malaria causes nearly 250 times more deaths in the world's poorest countries than in the richest. The economic burden of malaria to households can be extremely high. Even in the poor countries of sub-Saharan Africa, households have been found to spend between $2 and $25 on malaria treatment, and between $0.20 and $15 on prevention each month *(1)*. Treatment costs of malaria for small farmers have been estimated to be as high as 5% of total household expenditure in Kenya and 13% in Nigeria. Many are simply too poor to be able to pay for adequate protection.

Government resources are also stretched in the provision of prevention and treatment services. Between 20% and 40% of outpatient visits and between 10% and 15% of hospital admissions in Africa are attributed to malaria, at an estimated cost of $1.10 per outpatient visit (Malawi) and $35 per admission (Kenya). In Rwanda nearly a fifth of the health budget was spent on malaria treatment in 1989. One estimate of the impact of malaria on national income in Africa *(2)* put the economic burden at 0.6–1.0% of gross domestic product (GDP); separate estimates for Kenya put the overall production loss at 2–6% of GDP, and at 1–5% for Nigeria *(3)*.

Recent research *(4)* suggests that the adverse economic impact of malaria in Africa is probably even greater than 1% of GDP. This figure is mainly made up of estimated productivity losses through premature mortality and spells of sickness. Further, malaria in schoolchildren is a major cause of absenteeism and probably reduces the effectiveness of their education. It is also thought to drive away potential development opportunities by making certain zones unsuitable for habitation, deterring international trade and foreign investment, and jeopardizing the development of sectors such as tourism. Economic development may also be retarded by reduced access to international flows of knowledge and technology because companies may be reluctant to send representatives to malarious countries. Malaria may thus be a cause, and not just a consequence, of underdevelopment.

THE DIVERSE AND CHANGING NATURE OF THE DISEASE

The endemicity of malaria is largely dependent on the type of mosquito, the parasite species, and the climate, which broadly determine the intensity and length of transmission. Figure 4.1 shows malaria risk levels across sub-Saharan Africa *(5)*. Of the four species of parasite that affect humans, *Plasmodium falciparum* is the most dangerous. It is also the parasite most common in Africa. Epidemic areas are subject to irregular rapid increases in incidence, usually related to the season and population movements, whereas in endemic areas malaria transmission occurs continuously over many successive years. Endemic malaria under very high intensities of transmission, commonly referred to as stable endemic malaria, primarily exists in tropical Africa (except in highland areas) and in Papua New Guinea. Moderate intensities of transmission with seasonal and year to year fluctuations, referred to as unstable endemic malaria, prevails in much of the rest of the malaria world, particularly in Asia and Central and South America. Epidemics of malaria can also occur over large parts of the Indian peninsula, Sri Lanka, parts of the Middle East, South-East Asia, north-west Africa and some countries in South America. In highly endemic areas, children and pregnant women are the most vulnerable to attack, as other adults acquire a degree of immunity through continued exposure. But in areas of less intense transmission

Figure 4.1 Malaria risk across sub-Saharan Africa according to population density and climate [a]

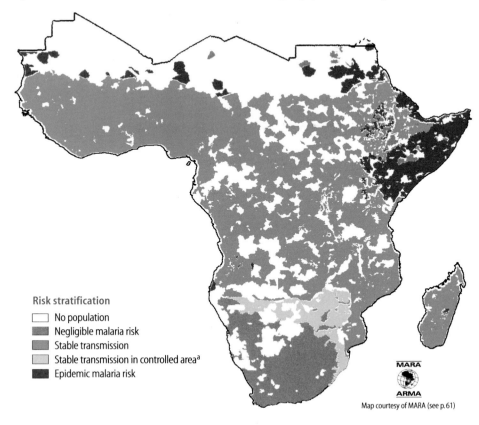

Risk stratification
☐ No population
▨ Negligible malaria risk
▨ Stable transmission
▨ Stable transmission in controlled area[a]
■ Epidemic malaria risk

MARA
ARMA
Map courtesy of MARA (see p. 61)

[a] Modelled on estimates of population density and stable transmission (transmission and/or new clinical cases every year), according to combined temperature and rainfall. In addition, in southern Africa, the fact that there has been a successful control strategy for many years was also taken into account.

Source: **Snow RW et al.** *Mortality, morbidity and disability due to malaria: A review of the African literature.* Report prepared for the Epidemiology & Burden of Disease Programme and Roll Back Malaria. Geneva, World Health Organization, 1998.

and particularly in epidemic areas, most of the population is likely to be non-immune and all are at risk.

The toll in morbidity and mortality from malaria has been held in check by the widespread availability of cheap and effective antimalarial drugs. The greatest threat to the control of malaria in the near future is the loss of effectiveness of these drugs because of resistance. The potentially lethal malaria parasite, *P. falciparum*, has shown itself capable of developing resistance to nearly all the antimalarial drugs now used. Chloroquine, perhaps the best ever antimalarial drug, and certainly the most widely used, is now failing against falciparum malaria in most areas of the tropical world.

In some areas, such as parts of South-East Asia and South America, chloroquine is now completely ineffective against *P. falciparum* malaria. In many parts of India and Africa, its effectiveness is falling rapidly. Even *Plasmodium vivax* malaria, which has been consistently sensitive to chloroquine in the past, has now developed resistance in some parts of South-East Asia and Oceania.

For the treatment of falciparum malaria, the usual successor to chloroquine is a combination of pyrimethamine and a long acting sulphonamide (SP), which is also affordable and well tolerated. Five countries in Africa (Botswana, Kenya, Malawi, South Africa and Swaziland) have now been forced to switch from chloroquine to SP as the first line antimalarial treatment. Unfortunately, in several of the areas where it has been deployed, notably South-East Asia and South America, *P. falciparum* has become widely SP-resistant.

Replacement drugs generally last only a few years before they too experience significant resistance. In some areas, such as Brazil and Thailand, only multi-drug therapies are now effective. Deciding when to change drugs is an extremely difficult decision, involving complex trade-offs between higher drug costs, immediate reductions in morbidity and mortality, reductions in the associated cost of treatment, and potential increases in resistance to replacement drugs, which could lead to higher morbidity and mortality in the future. Policymakers urgently need good data and practical advice to help them to choose the most appropriate drug regimen. Policies must be developed to balance the need for accessible treatment with the need to control drug use in order to reduce the growth in resistance.

Human beings play a crucial role in the epidemiology of malaria. Epidemics can result from population movement of non-immunes into malarious areas, either in search of temporary work, or into new frontier settlements, for example in jungle areas of South America, or as refugees, following natural disaster, war or civil unrest. Nchinda *(6)* cites armed conflict and migration as important causes of malaria resurgence in Africa. Economic activity and development can create conditions suitable for mosquito breeding through, for example, environmental changes such as deforestation, global warming and irrigation. Furthermore, previous patterns of antimalarial and insecticide use affect present levels of drug and insecticide resistance.

MALARIA CONTROL: PAST, PRESENT AND FUTURE

The nature of malaria and its impact on health is quite different in different places. So control operations must be specific to each location and need to take into account the epidemiological, economic, institutional and cultural settings. Patterns of promotive and preventive behaviour, and of treatment seeking, are influenced by levels of education and cultural beliefs. And the capacity to control both the disease and the growth of resistance depends on the quality and coverage of each country's general infrastructure and the state of its health system.

CONTROL STRATEGIES, 1950–1990s

Organized efforts to reduce the burden of malaria can be traced back to antiquity, and a historical perspective offers important insights into control strategies (see Box 4.2). In the postwar period several distinct shifts have occurred in global and national strategies to control malaria, reflecting changing attitudes to disease control in general and growing knowledge about malaria in particular.

The period from the late 1940s to the mid-1960s was a time of optimism. Following the discovery of DDT and the establishment of the World Health Organization, malaria eradication was identified as a priority. Time limited special-purpose campaigns, involving DDT spraying, chloroquine chemotherapy and active case surveillance, were expected to achieve global eradication in a matter of years. "This is the DDT era of malariology. For the first time it is economically feasible for nations, however undeveloped and whatever the climate, to banish malaria completely from their borders" wrote one authority in 1955 *(7)*. Cases of malaria fell dramatically in several countries, most notably in Sri Lanka (see Box 4.1), where they dropped from over one million cases a year to under twenty in 1963. But resistance developed to DDT, and concerns about its safety emerged. External funding was scaled back, and public support for spraying wavered. By 1969, WHO had accepted that control programmes were indispensable in areas where eradication was impractical, such as sub-Saharan Africa (where eradication strategies were never attempted), and early optimism was giving way to disillusion.

International funding for malaria control and research shrank in the 1970s and 1980s, and the emphasis shifted to control strategies. But there were no clear guidelines, and many malaria programmes, set up originally as "one-off" eradication campaigns, were organizationally outside the rest of the health system. Resistance to chloroquine grew rapidly, first in Asia, subsequently in Africa. Major epidemics occurred in Brazil (1985–1989), India (1974–1977) and Turkey (1976–1978).

Although global malaria eradication was not achieved, gains were made, and important lessons were learned from the experience of the 1950s and 1960s. First, malaria was eradi-

---

Box 4.2 Malaria control: lessons from the past

Organized efforts to reduce the burden of malaria are as old as human societies. From the time of the pre-Roman Etruscans to Napoleon, for example, efforts were made to drain the marshes surrounding Rome, whose "noisome smells" were believed to cause pestilence (7). Hippocrates observed that "[where] there be rivers ... which drain off from the ground the stagnant water ... [the people] will be healthy and bright. But if there be no rivers, and the water that the people drink be marshy ... the physique of the people must show protruding bellies and enlarged spleens". Before the parasites were discovered and their life cycle characterized, malaria could only be associated with poor sanitation. Accordingly, therefore, most early efforts at malaria control focused on sanitation and land use strategy.

The expansion of colonial powers into the malarious tropics brought new urgency to European efforts to understand the etiology of malaria. Throughout the 19th century, a succession of colonial army officers, as well as scientists from Italy (which was malaria-endemic at the time), doggedly tracked the disease until its entire life cycle, etiology, and epidemiology had been elucidated in

detail. When Ronald Ross provided irrefutable empirical support for the mosquito theory, malaria intervention became aimed at reducing vector populations.

In addition to spurring the development of modern malariology, the increase of global traffic during the colonial period resulted in the importation of many infectious diseases to areas where they had not previously been endemic. Malaria, for example, was imported into Mauritius in 1866. Similar introductions of malaria occurred at the same time on Grand Comoros Island and Reunion Island. Malaria remained endemic in Mauritius and Reunion for a century before it was sustainably controlled.

By the time of the outbreak of the First World War, emerging success stories in Panama and southern Europe and unsuccessful attempts elsewhere spawned debates which would shape later international policies to control malaria transmission. Among these debates, the alternative conceptions of malaria as a social disease – to be solved by the elimination of poverty – and as an entomological and clinical problem which required proper scientific intervention strategy vied with each other for decades. Ultimately, the discovery of DDT's unprecedented insecticidal potential would infuse new

energy into vector-based approaches to malaria control.

The two World Wars, with their concomitant social upheaval, transformed anti-malaria efforts around the world. In the rural south of the United States and in southern Europe the prevalence of malaria had begun to decline. This was mainly attributable to the interplay between malaria transmission dynamics specific to these regions and to three important changes attendant on rapid economic growth.

- The drainage of swamps in order to establish new agricultural land had drastically reduced the indigenous anopheline populations of malaria endemic regions. Similarly, improved facilities in animal husbandry led to better separation of humans and livestock, and diverted the attention of more zoophilic vectors.
- Increased income provided at-risk individuals with the means to improve their health-seeking behaviour, including limiting their exposure to mosquitoes and seeking drug treatment. Many radical malaria treatment strategies aim not only to eliminate clinical symptoms of the disease but also to clear all parasites from the patient's blood. Similarly, increased national wealth allowed for the establishment of an

extensive health infrastructure, making primary clinical care easily accessible. Malaria was relatively easy to diagnose in these regions, where it was one of only a few vector-borne infectious diseases.

- The establishment of large cities created environments hostile to the spread of malaria.

Analysis of historical changes in malaria prevalence suggests a number of factors which help to determine the likelihood and sustainability of success in malaria control. Among these are geography, evolutionary history of flora and fauna, infrastructure, and land use. It is due to these factors, much more than to socioeconomic ones, that attempts to control or interrupt transmission of the disease have historically been most successful on islands, in temperate climates, or at high elevations. These lessons have important policy implications for malaria control; well-designed strategies ought to consider how such factors interact both locally and globally. Interventions must be critically assessed to ensure that they are suited to the geographical, economic and biological contexts in which they are carried out.

Contributed by Amar Hamoudi & Jeffrey D. Sachs, Harvard Institute for International Development, Cambridge MA, USA.

cated or controlled in ecological zones where infection was lower: in the many subtropical areas of southern Europe, the island settings of Mauritius and Singapore, in Hong Kong (China), and also in parts of Malaysia. Second, the importance of supportive health systems to malaria control efforts became clear. Sri Lanka came close to eradication in large part because of its well-organized and accessible health system.

By 1992, when a revised global malaria control strategy was approved by WHO's Member States at the World Health Assembly, there had been much re-thinking. Resistance had spread but new drugs and tools were becoming available. Malaria control was recognized to be an essential part of overall health development, and the importance of achieving sustainable progress was emphasized. National programmes were encouraged to focus on early diagnosis and prompt treatment, selective and sustainable prevention, early detection, containment and prevention of epidemics, and building local capacity to assess and manage the malaria situation. In Brazil, a control programme integrated within the health system rapidly expanded diagnostic and treatment facilities between 1992 and 1996 and achieved a substantial reduction in *P. falciparum* malaria transmission. Africa, the most affected region, took important initiatives (see Box 4.3). Mobilization of the research community was achieved with the launch of the Multilateral Initiative on Malaria in 1997.

CURRENT TECHNOLOGY FOR EFFECTIVE INTERVENTIONS

A wide range of effective tools for malaria prevention is at present available, though not always where most needed.

- Insecticide-treated nets have increasingly been used over the last 15 years as a method of preventing mosquito biting. Where nets are already widely used in the community, only a re-impregnation programme is required; but where net ownership is currently low, nets must also be distributed as part of the intervention. Large-scale use of insecticide-treated nets has been accompanied by substantial reductions in malaria incidence in China and Viet Nam. The use of treated bednets and curtains has led to reductions in child mortality ranging from 14% to 63% in African trials, but current implementation in Africa remains limited and achieving high retreatment rates of nets has proved very difficult. Nets are not a panacea.

Box 4.3 Malaria control in Africa

Malaria is the leading health problem in sub-Saharan Africa, where 74% of the population live in highly endemic areas and a further 18% live in epidemic areas. About 550 million people are at risk of malaria. There are about 270 million cases a year, with almost one million deaths; 5% of children are likely to die of malaria-related illness before they are five years old.

Malaria has spread into areas which previously had low transmission or none at all. For example, epidemics have occurred in recent years in some parts of eastern and southern Africa. This changing geographical distribution is influenced by population movements, as well as by global warming and deteriorating sanitation which make the environment more propitious for the breeding of mosquitos.

Countries in the African region have adopted a coordinated malaria control strategy which includes: the early detection, control or prevention of epidemics; early diagnosis of malaria cases, with prompt and effective treatment; preventive measures including vector control activities; and integration of activities into primary health care.

Over the past two years, capacity has been built in the areas of policy formulation, the planning and evaluation of malaria control programmes, and case management at all levels of the health system including the community. A review of health facilities in selected districts found that, in general, the quality of case management is improving. Uncomplicated cases of malaria were being correctly managed in 67–100% of health facilities and severe malaria in 28–100%. Preventive measures, such as indoor spraying, personal protection and the use of bednets, are being promoted.

Priorities for malaria control in Africa are now the strengthening of technical support to programmes, training, and enhanced operational research. Countries will be encouraged to build partnerships for the systematic implementation of the malaria control strategy, and communities will be encouraged to play a greater role.

Contributed by the WHO Regional Office for Africa.

- User-friendly packaging of drugs is a simple and cost-effective way to improve case management and compliance. Better regulation of drug vendors, which is also necessary, presents a bigger challenge.
- Access to early treatment of good quality remains a critical need. Effective treatment of African children could bring about an immediate reduction in the total disease burden. Chemoprophylaxis or presumptive treatment during pregnancy reduces the risk of malaria infection in all pregnant women and significantly increases the birth weight of babies born to women in their first pregnancy. Although WHO recommends that all pregnant women in malaria endemic areas receive regular prophylaxis, in practice less than 20% of women are effectively covered. For both women and children at risk from malaria, better functioning health systems have an important potential role.
- Using a stratified approach to residual house spraying and applying it in high-risk areas remains an important control activity in many countries. Larvicides or environmental management, such as drainage or control of water flow of rivers and other water bodies, can be used to destroy mosquito larvae, but only in areas where breeding sites are well defined.

For an intervention to be appropriate it must not only be effective but also cost-effective compared with alternative uses of scarce resources. The cost-effectiveness of each intervention will vary, depending on epidemiological factors (such as the length of transmission season), economic variables (such as local costs for staff, nets and drugs), and behavioural factors (such as adherence to drug regimens and retreatment rates for nets). The extent and quality of the existing health infrastructure is also a key factor in determining costs and cost-effectiveness. For example, the cost-effectiveness of insecticide-treated nets varies according to whether nets are available in the community, and the cost-effectiveness of presumptive treatment in pregnancy depends on whether there is already wide coverage of antenatal care.

Figure 4.2 shows the range of the cost per DALY averted by preventive strategies in poor areas of Africa with high levels of malaria transmission *(8)*. It also shows estimates (from different sources) of the cost per DALY averted from improved treatment interventions. It is possible to make rough comparisons with data for other health interventions, although the methodologies used may not be strictly comparable. For example, the cost-effectiveness of measles vaccination is between $2 and $17 per DALY averted, onchocerciasis vector control between $120 and $230, and the medical management of hypertension greater than $2000, converted to 1995 US$ *(9)*. The Brazilian national malaria control programme, with a mix of vector control and integrated early diagnosis and treatment, reduced the burden of malaria at an estimated cost of $65 per DALY averted. It has recently been argued that any interventions with a cost per DALY averted of less than $150 would count as cost-effective in low income countries. Compared with this threshold, all the malaria control interventions evaluated represent good value for money. These data are consistent with a cost per death avoided of between $750 and $2500. On this basis, the annual global cost of halving malaria deaths would be between $375 million and $1.25 billion.

Effective, low technology interventions can be used to improve the quality of case management, even in the presence of considerable drug resistance. The development of simple algorithms improves diagnosis, increased drug testing can help identify poor quality antimalarials, and training of providers in both the public and private sectors is needed to improve prescription practices. Providing simple instructions and pre-packaging drugs help to ensure that the correct course of treatment is taken, and the identification of severe cases

Figure 4.2 Comparative cost-effectiveness of selected malaria control interventions in a typical low income African country, US$, 1995

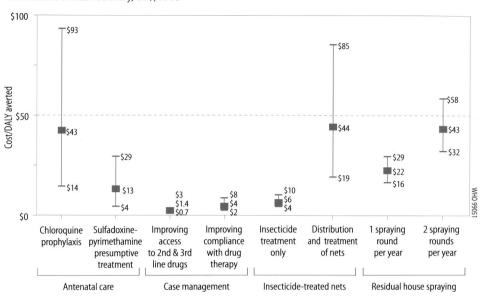

The following assumptions are made:
  – antenatal care: primigravidae only, 50% chloroquine RII/RIII resistance, 10% sulfadoxine-pyrimethamine RII/RIII resistance;
  – case management: gross costs, chloroquine as first line drug with 30% clinical failure;
  – insecticide-treated nets: one treatment of deltamethrin a year, no insecticide resistance;
  – residual house spraying: lambda-cyhalothrin, no insecticide resistance.
Adapted from: **Goodman CA, Coleman PG, Mills A.** *Economic analysis of malaria control in sub-Saharan Africa.* Report to Global Forum for
  Health Research. London, London School of Hygiene and Tropical Medicine (Health Economics and Financing Programme), 1998.

can be improved by community-wide health education. Where resistance is high, health outcomes can be improved by ensuring that treatment failures are recognized and treated with appropriate second line drugs. Although data are limited, several of these interventions are potentially highly cost-effective. For example, based on a situation of 30% clinical failure with chloroquine as first line drug, the cost per DALY averted of improving adherence through pre-packaging and education is likely to be under $8 in low income African countries, and improving the availability of second and third line drugs can cost less than $3 per DALY averted. Both interventions would be affordable to low income countries, requiring less than a 0.5% addition to the existing health sector budget.

An intervention can be cost-effective but also very expensive. Figure 4.3 shows the cost of implementing the different preventive and treatment interventions, as a percentage of the public sector health budget for a typical low income African country *(8)*. The results are striking. Whilst antenatal presumptive treatment and insecticide treatment of existing nets are both relatively inexpensive, distributing and treating nets on a national scale would require a budget increase of nearly 25%, and country-wide residual spraying would increase the budget by over 50%. These amounts are unaffordable to low income countries through government finance alone.

The focusing of public resources on a limited number of highly effective, low cost interventions will include preventive and promotive actions, and treatment of malaria. For example, the Integrated Management of Childhood Illness (IMCI) package is an initiative to improve the treatment of the most common childhood diseases and conditions. Malaria is one of five key conditions included in the strategy, along with acute respiratory infections,

Figure 4.3 Comparative affordability of selected malaria control interventions: total cost of full coverage as a percentage of a public sector health budget for a typical low income African country

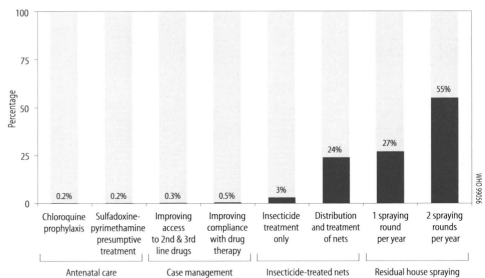

The following assumptions are made:
  – antenatal care: primigravidae only, 50% chloroquine RII/RIII resistance, 10% sulfadoxine-pyrimethamine RII/RIII resistance;
  – case management: gross costs, chloroquine as first line drug with 30% clinical failure;
  – insecticide-treated nets: one treatment of deltamethrin a year, no insecticide resistance;
  – residual house spraying: lambda-cyhalothrin, no insecticide resistance.
Adapted from: **Goodman CA, Coleman PG, Mills A.** *Economic analysis of malaria control in sub-Saharan Africa.* Report to Global Forum for Health Research. London, London School of Hygiene and Tropical Medicine (Health Economics and Financing Programme), 1998.

measles, diarrhoea and malnutrition. Integrated management involves the training of health care staff and the provision of guidelines to help health care providers to recognize the considerable overlap in the signs and symptoms of these common diseases, and to encourage prevention and appropriate treatment of children at home and in the health facility.

Preliminary estimates suggest that, in sub-Saharan Africa alone, IMCI could avert annually over 400 000 deaths due to malaria in children. In addition, IMCI could avert a further 350 000 childhood deaths from other causes in sub-Saharan Africa and perhaps five times this number globally. In the *World development report 1993*, the World Bank estimated the annual average cost of IMCI implementation at US$ 30–50 per DALY averted. This puts IMCI in the middle range of the interventions presented in Figure 4.2. However, the absolute impact of IMCI on disease burden would be considerably greater than that of most of the interventions shown. WHO is conducting a multi-country evaluation of IMCI effectiveness in order to provide more accurate figures.

Past experience has demonstrated that, although all of these strategies provide promising opportunities for improving the quality of care, their success will depend on integration with, and development of, existing primary health care activities, and the strengthening of health care services in general.

FUTURE CONTROL STRATEGIES AND RESEARCH NEEDS

The provision of prompt diagnosis and effective treatment should be a key component of any control programme, but in reality disease management is often grossly inadequate. This reflects a general weakness in the availability and quality of existing health systems.

A clear lesson from past experience of malaria control is that both prevention and treatment need to be delivered through a strong health system. Separate malaria organizations are not sustainable entities, and their effect has been to detract resources and attention from securing health system improvement and reform. Often, access to skilled care providers is impossible. Poor people face both price and time barriers in accessing health care. At first levels of care, providers may prescribe inappropriate drugs, patients may not comply with the recommended regimen, drugs are often ineffective because of resistance or poor quality, and patients with severe malaria are misdiagnosed or fail to get specialist care. Inadequate care results in unnecessary morbidity and mortality from malaria, and also encourages the development of drug resistance through the use of suboptimal doses.

Malaria control in the 21st century will be approached through strengthened health systems, working closely with local communities to identify and tackle the specific problems of the area. An impressive array of tools for preventive and effective treatment is already available. Big inroads can be made into malaria morbidity and mortality. The nine most endemic countries in the region of the Americas achieved a 60% reduction in malaria mortality between 1994 and 1997. Even with growing resistance, an estimated 20% reduction in child deaths in Africa could be achieved if health systems were funded, organized and managed to bring today's knowledge and techniques within the reach of whole populations. The state of the health system in most poor countries is itself a contributor to the scale of the malaria problem. Applying available knowledge is a prerequisite to future progress.

The Multilateral Initiative on Malaria in Africa (see Box 4.4) was created in 1997 to boost collaboration in malaria research to support strategies for control. The initiative aims to increase the funding for research on malaria (by one estimate currently just over 1% of the research funding level for HIV/AIDS) and bring together scientists, funding agencies, the pharmaceutical industry and government to identify common research priorities. Another joint public–private sector initiative is the Medicines for Malaria Venture (MMV) which aims to develop anti-malarial drugs and drug combinations and make them available in poor countries. Support for this venture is being solicited from foundations and other public sources as well as from the pharmaceutical industry.

Drugs, such as mefloquine, are now available, which are effective against multi-resistant falciparum malaria. But there are two problems; the first is that they are expensive and may cost 5–10 times as much per treatment as the drug they are succeeding. The second problem is that resistance can develop to these drugs, too. Artemisinin and its derivatives have proved the most rapidly acting and potent of all antimalarials. In large clinical trials these compounds have proved safe and effective, both in severe and uncomplicated malaria. The

---

Box 4.4 Multilateral Initiative on Malaria in Africa

The Multilateral Initiative on Malaria (MIM) was launched in Dakar, Senegal, in January 1997 when a number of institutions from both the public and private sectors joined forces to promote malaria research in Africa. In the context of this Initiative, the UNDP/World Bank/WHO Special Programme for Research and Training in Tropical Diseases is coordinating a Task Force on Malaria Research Capability Strengthening in Africa, which will focus on the needs of endemic countries and fund activities related to strengthening research capacities in malaria. A budget of about US$ 3 million a year has been raised, with contributions from several institutions to support research and capacity-building projects and training.

The Task Force has mobilized over 40 countries and 160 partners to submit proposals for review. Fifteen partnership projects involving 20 African and 5 European countries and the USA have so far been funded, and 14 research training grants have been approved in connection with the projects. The main research areas to be funded are antimalarial drug policy and chemotherapy, epidemiology, pathogenesis, vectors, and health systems and social science.

use of these drugs in combinations may provide an answer to the seemingly inexorable increase in resistance. Investigating this possibility is a major research priority. Combining artemisinin derivatives with mefloquine has been shown to halt the increase in mefloquine resistance on the western border of Thailand. Rational and appropriate use of these antimalarial drug combinations will require a concerted effort to educate medical personnel, dispensers, traditional healers and people living in endemic areas on the appropriate use of antimalarial drugs.

But malaria control is not exclusively a challenge of implementation. New knowledge, products and tools are urgently needed. In particular, new drugs are required. Investment in vaccine development now has a high probability of success. This and other discoveries in molecular genetics require political and financial guarantees to sustain their development into usable products, which the Multilateral Initiative on Malaria is working to secure. And careful economic and epidemiological research is needed to ensure that the most cost-effective mix of promotive, preventive and treatment actions is implemented to meet the needs of defined populations.

The versatility and adaptability of malaria pose a serious threat to successful control. This is particularly true in situations of war and social turmoil or of rapid environmental change. Over the last few years, several new and innovative products and strategies have become available and several others are at an advanced stage of development (see Box 4.5).

- Promising results have been achieved in early trials of suppositories containing the fast acting antimalarial, artesunate. Artesunate suppositories can be given to patients referred to hospital with severe malaria, who are unable to take oral medication. By allowing the rapid administration of an effective antimalarial their chance of survival both during transport and in hospital should be improved.

- New dipstick tests for diagnosing malaria are now on the market. The tests are quick and do not require sophisticated laboratory skills, equipment or an electricity supply. At over $1 per test, widescale use in Africa is unlikely to be affordable, but the tests could be cost-effective in improving the diagnostic accuracy in areas where expensive first line drugs such as mefloquine are used, or in the early confirmation of suspected epidemics.

- Combination therapies designed to slow the development of drug resistance are currently being tested. If two drugs are used together, the chance that a mutant will emerge

---

Box 4.5 Malaria vaccine development

The development of an effective vaccine is the major breakthrough needed in malaria control. Even with much lower efficacy than other vaccines, a malaria vaccine is likely to be hugely cost-effective. Progress in understanding the immune mechanisms involved in conferring protection against malaria, and in identifying vaccine candidates and their genes, has been substantial. Vaccine development is now at a point of unprecedented opportunity, though it may take 7–15 years before an effective vaccine is ready.

Several different approaches to a malaria vaccine, using the latest advances in technology, are undergoing field testing on volunteers in Africa, Asia and the United States. The whole genome (the complete set of hereditary factors) of the malaria parasite is being sequenced.

Asexual blood stage vaccines, based on cocktails of antigens, have already been tested. Spf66, a synthetic peptide vaccine developed by Manuel Pattaroyo in the Instituto de Inmunología in Bogotá, Colombia, has been only partially effective in field tri-

als in South America, South-East Asia and Africa. Sophisticated biochemical methods are now being used to improve its potency.

A project taking advantage of DNA research is MuStDO 15.1 (multi-stage vaccine operation), a 15-gene malaria DNA vaccine designed to reduce morbidity and mortality in young children in sub-Saharan Africa. It is expected to enter clinical trials in the year 2000.

Already in field trials in the Gambia, a recombinant protein vaccine, RTS S, developed by SmithKline Biologicals, is designed to prevent the malaria

parasite infectious stage from entering or developing within human liver cells. Vaccines such as this will prevent the life-threatening consequences of malaria in non-immune individuals.

A different approach is a vaccine that prevents the transmission of the malaria parasite from an infected person to another. A transmission blocking vaccine is under development by scientists at the United States National Institutes of Health, in collaboration with WHO.

that is simultaneously resistant to both drugs is much lower than if the drugs are used alone. This strategy would increase drug costs in the short run, but could be highly beneficial if the useful life of available antimalarials is prolonged.

- For insecticide-treated nets, "dip-it-yourself" insecticide treatment kits are under development. These kits can be used in the home and should make retreatment more convenient. Social marketing strategies can be used to promote the use of treated nets.

Progress in the development of computer-based information systems allows geographical data to be combined with information on climate, environment, drug and pesticide resistance, population size and the location of health services. An example is MARA (Mapping Malaria Risk in Africa International Collaboration), an initiative to map malaria risk according to epidemiological type, which will provide vital information for assessing the disease burden and planning control. Information on the costs of malaria control, and how these vary by location and the scale of the intervention, is essential for the evaluation of both the cost-effectiveness and affordability of strategies. Operational research is necessary to devise ways to implement strategies which are sustainable and locally acceptable. Health services in general must be strengthened to provide a firm base for the delivery of malaria prevention and treatment, and new control strategies must be integrated within the national health care system.

A Global Programme to Roll Back Malaria

Several forces have combined to bring about the resurgence of malaria: civil conflict and large-scale human migrations, climatic and environmental change, inadequate and deteriorating health systems, and growing insecticide and drug resistance. For the following reasons, a new global initiative is timely.

- Malaria is a major problem. Although existing data are inadequate, it is clear that the level of the health burden of malaria, and its heavy incidence on the poorest populations, make it a powerful debilitating force.
- Tackling malaria is thus a major battle in the war against poverty. Malaria is a social and economic development issue, not just a health concern.
- Successful malaria control involves strengthening health systems. Weak health systems and uninvolved communities are part of the malaria problem. Because malaria is an acute condition with a rapid natural history, easy access to health care of good quality is vital in its management. Externally driven initiatives, by-passing local and national health systems, are neither sustainable nor supportive to malaria control and health development. Many countries have begun the process of reforming their health systems to improve performance. Malaria control, like the better management of all illnesses, needs to build on and support these changes. Through strengthened health systems, total malaria deaths could be halved for about $1 billion per year.
- A willingness to collaborate has been demonstrated. The Organization of African Unity, the World Bank and WHO's African Region have already planned a major African Malaria Initiative which is expected to spearhead Roll Back Malaria. The Multilateral Initiative on Malaria is under way, and a new alliance between public and private sectors in the form of the Medicines for Malaria Venture has been set up, aiming to improve the availability of effective antimalarials in poor countries.

Roll Back Malaria is different from previous efforts to fight malaria. It will work through new tools for controlling malaria, but also by strengthening health systems for sustainable health improvement. Roll Back Malaria's activities will be implemented through partnerships with international organizations, governments in endemic and non-endemic countries, academic institutions, the private sector and nongovernmental organizations (see Box 4.6). As agreed in October 1998, it will be supported by the united efforts of the four international agencies most concerned with malaria and its effects on health and the economy: UNICEF, the United Nations Development Programme, the World Bank and the World Health Organization.

Roll Back Malaria will act as a pathfinder, helping to set the direction and strategy for more integrated action in other priority areas such as tuberculosis control and safe motherhood. Greater reliance on partnerships in fighting malaria will inform WHO's approach to other major health challenges, and the development of effective and coordinated multipartner action.

Though the disease burden from malaria is still very high, the situation has improved greatly since the beginning of the century. Trends in Africa are a conspicuous exception.

Since the beginning of the 1990s, a new international solidarity has arisen for renewal of the combat against malaria.

A major challenge is to optimize the use of available tools to deal with the disease, in coordination with all partners involved, through strengthened health systems; and to make a big step forward in research in the areas of vaccines and drugs.

Box 4.6 How Roll Back Malaria will operate

Governments and civil society in malaria-affected countries will take the lead in Roll Back Malaria (RBM) as a means to reduce poverty and mortality, and promote human development. UN system agencies will work with them: WHO, the World Bank, UNDP and UNICEF are committed partners. Other partners in the international initiative will include bilateral agencies, foundations, nongovernmental organizations, private sector entities (particularly research-based pharmaceutical companies) and the media. Partners will work together, at country level, towards common goals using agreed strategies and procedures. Usually the country's national authorities will direct the partnership.

Once a country has committed itself to the RBM initiative, it will undertake a situation analysis so

partners can develop a strategy for intensified action against malaria. Partners will agree interventions for each location after examining information about the extent to which people prevent themselves from getting malaria; treat themselves when ill with malaria; and have access to good quality health care.

Partners will also consider health sector issues – particularly the institutional and financial context within which health care is being offered and used, both in the public and private sectors.

WHO has established a Cabinet project to help country RBM partnerships become fully effective. It supports them by:

• endorsing the technical content of strategies being pursued by partners;

• brokering technical and financial assistance for their implementation;

• encouraging partners to stick to their agreements;

• monitoring progress in rolling back malaria, within the context of health sector development.

To provide countries with the specialized technical support they need in tackling malaria, the project will sponsor a number of resource networks (initially a dozen), each concerned with a specific issue, such as avoiding resistance to antimalarial medication or insecticides. Networks will be made up of experts in the appropriate field – particularly from the relevant region. They will encourage collaboration between countries, will link malaria control teams with researchers and will optimize the use of local expertise in the management of malaria control activities. This will enable implementation plans to reflect an evidence-based response to local needs and

realities, in keeping with the Global Strategy for Malaria Control adopted in Amsterdam in 1992.

The project promotes effective investment in new medicines, vaccines and other tools to reduce malaria-related suffering through the Multilateral Research Initiative on Malaria and the public–private Medicines for Malaria Venture.

The project helps increase the level of international financial investment in countries' efforts to roll back malaria, through international advocacy with an emphasis on the current and potential investment outcomes – particularly among members of the global RBM partnership. The project will also ensure up-to-date aggregation and analysis of information on the global malaria situation.

REFERENCES

1. **Chima RI, Mills A.** *Estimating the economic impact of malaria in sub-Saharan Africa: A review of the evidence.* London, London School of Hygiene and Tropical Medicine, 1998 (mimeographed document).

2. **Shepard DS et al.** The economic cost of malaria in Africa. *Tropical medicine and parasitology,* 1991, **42**: 199–203.

3. **Leighton C, Foster R.** *Economic impacts of malaria in Kenya and Nigeria.* Bethesda MD, Abt Associates, 1993, Major applied research paper no. 6, Health financing and sustainability project.

4. **Bloom DE, Sachs JD.** Geography, demography, and economic growth in Africa. *Brookings papers on economic activity,* 1998, **2**:207–295.

5. **Snow RW et al.** *Mortality, morbidity and disability due to malaria: A review of the African literature.* Report prepared for the Epidemiology & Burden of Disease Programme and Roll Back Malaria. Geneva, World Health Organization, 1998.

6. **Nchinda TC.** Malaria, a re-emerging disease in Africa. *Emerging infectious diseases,* 1998, **4**(3): 398–403.

7. **Russell PF.** *Man's mastery over malaria.* London, Oxford University Press, 1955.

8. **Goodman CA, Coleman PG, Mills A.** *Economic analysis of malaria control in sub-Saharan Africa.* Report to Global Forum for Health Research. London, London School of Hygiene and Tropical Medicine (Health Economics and Financing Programme), 1998.

9. **Jamison D et al (eds).** *Disease control priorities in developing countries.* New York, Oxford University Press for The World Bank, 1993.

5

COMBATING THE

TOBACCO EPIDEMIC

*W*ith current smoking patterns, about 500 million people alive today will eventually be killed by tobacco *(1)*. Tobacco deaths will occur in men already smoking, children who will become smokers, and an increasing number of women smokers. For most of these deaths to be avoided, a substantial proportion of adult smokers will have to quit and children will need to avoid taking up the habit. If half of the adult smokers stopped over the next 20 years, about one third of the tobacco deaths in 2020 would be avoided and tobacco deaths in the second quarter of the century would be halved. Such changes would avoid about 20 or 30 million tobacco deaths in the first quarter of the century and about 140 million in the second quarter (see Figure 5.1).

How can the epidemic be fought? Effective tobacco control strategies already exist, and they have been proved to make a difference, benefiting both adults and children. Governments that have adopted them have succeeded in reducing, or at least slowing the increase in, tobacco use.

To build on those successes, four principles of tobacco control provide a road-map for national and global action. They include public health information combined with advertising bans, taxes and regulations, encouraging smoking cessation, and building tobacco control coalitions. They are described in detail later in this chapter.

This chapter also reviews the health and economic costs of tobacco, and identifies major obstacles that control programmes must overcome. It looks at what has and has not worked, and shows that the tools for control exist. The lack of global leadership has, however, resulted in the potential for worldwide control remaining unrealized. The final section of this chapter explains how WHO's Tobacco Free Initiative (TFI) aims to fill the gap in leadership.

THE HEALTH AND ECONOMIC COSTS
OF TOBACCO USE

Worldwide mortality from tobacco is likely to rise from about four million deaths a year in 1998 to about 10 million a year in 2030. To put it slightly differently, tobacco will cause about 150 million deaths in the first quarter of the century and 300 million in the second quarter. Half of these deaths will occur in the 35–69 years age group, including many in productive middle age, with an average loss of 20–25 years of life.

Tobacco use results in both health and economic costs that are large and growing. This section summarizes the evidence.

HEALTH CONSEQUENCES OF TOBACCO

Since about 1950, more than 70 000 scientific articles have left no scientific doubt that prolonged smoking is an important cause of premature mortality and disability worldwide. Estimates suggest that in developed countries, smoking will have caused about 62 million deaths between 1950 and 2000. WHO now estimates that smoking causes about four million deaths annually worldwide (see Table 5.1) and predicts that, with current smoking patterns, this number is likely to increase dramatically.

There is, of course, some uncertainty in such estimates, both because they involve extrapolation of present hazards to future hazards, and because they involve extrapolation from studies in Western Europe, North America and China to many other populations. At present many large countries lack direct evidence on their tobacco mortality; in addition, the long delay between smoking and its mortality effects has confused governments and individuals. For example, while studies in the 1960s suggested that one in four long-term smokers died from their habit, studies in the 1990s suggest that the real ratio is now about one in two. In addition, those smokers dying between ages 35 and 69 lose about 20–25 years of life versus non-smoker life expectancy, and those dying over age 70 lose about 8 years of life.

The nature of the smoking epidemic also varies from country to country. In developed countries, cardiovascular disease, in particular ischaemic heart disease, is the most common smoking-related cause of death. In populations where cigarette smoking has been common for several decades, about 90% of lung cancer, 15–20% of other cancers, 75% of chronic bronchitis and emphysema, and 25% of deaths from cardiovascular disease at ages 35–69 years are attributable to tobacco. Tobacco-related cancer constitutes 16% of the total annual incidence of cancer cases – and 30% of cancer deaths – in developed countries, while the corresponding figure in developing countries is 10% (2). By contrast, in China, which has the world's highest number of tobacco deaths, smoking now causes far more deaths from chronic respiratory diseases than it does from cardiovascular disease. In addition, smoking causes about 12% of all tuberculosis deaths. Men in urban China smoking more than 20 cigarettes a day have double the death rate from TB of non-smokers. This could be because a lung damaged by tobacco may offer a propitious environment for the infectious tuberculosis bacillus.

Exposure to other people's smoking is associated with a somewhat higher risk of lung cancer, and with several other important health ailments in children such as sudden infant death syndrome, low birth weight, intrauterine growth retardation and children's respiratory disease. In addition, smoking is the leading cause of domestic fires in the United States, Canada and other high income countries, entailing billions of dollars of property loss annually.

Current deaths from tobacco relate to past consumption, mainly among males in developed countries and in

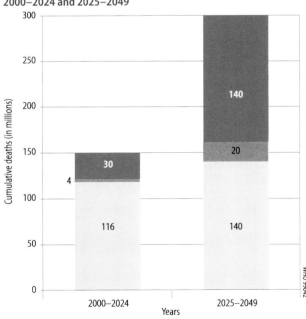

Figure 5.1 Premature deaths from tobacco use, projections for 2000–2024 and 2025–2049

Cumulative deaths (in millions)

WHO 99042

■ Preventable if adults quit (halving global cigarette consumption by 2020)
▨ Preventable if young adults do not start (halving global uptake of smoking by 2020)
□ Other premature deaths from tobacco-related causes

Source: *Background: Future world tobacco deaths.* Clinical Trial Service Unit and Epidemiological Studies Unit, University of Oxford, 1998.

China. In the near future, the epidemic will expand to include more developing countries and a larger number of women. Lung cancer is now the most common cause of death from cancer in women in the United States and its incidence in women is rising briskly in countries where female smoking is long established *(3)*.

The scale of the approaching epidemic can be gauged from the estimate that there are about 1.15 billion smokers in the world today, consuming an average of 14 cigarettes each per day *(4)*. Of these smokers, 82% live in low and middle income countries – a result, in part, of inadequate tobacco controls.

Tobacco consumption fell between 1981 and 1991 in most high income countries (see Figure 5.2). In the United States, the prevalence of smoking increased steadily from the 1930s and reached a peak in 1964 when more than 40% of all adult Americans, including 60% of men, smoked. Since then smoking prevalence has decreased, falling to 23% by 1997. By contrast, consumption is increasing in developing countries by about 3.4% per annum, having risen dramatically in some countries in recent years. Overall, smoking prevalence among men in developing countries is about 48%.

Thus, on current smoking patterns, by the third decade of the next century, smoking is expected to kill 10 million people annually worldwide – more than the total of deaths from malaria, maternal and major childhood conditions, and tuberculosis combined *(5)*. Over 70% of these deaths will be in the developing world. By 2020, smoking will cause about one in three of all adult deaths, up from one in six adult deaths in 1990 *(6)*.

Table 5.1 Tobacco: cigarette consumption, mortality and disease burden by WHO Region

WHO Region	Cigarette consumption per capita[a] estimates for around 1995	Mortality (000) estimates for 1998	DALYs (000) estimates for 1998
Africa	480	125	1 900
The Americas	1 530	582	6 787
Eastern Mediterranean	890	182	2 976
Europe	2 080	1 369	18 141
South-East Asia	415	580	7 439
Western Pacific	1 945	1 185	12 044
World total	1 325	4 023	49 288

[a] These figures exclude other tobacco products and may significantly underestimate tobacco consumption. Because of a change in methodology, comparison with previous WHO estimates should be avoided. Based on data from the UN Department for Economic and Social Information and Policy Analysis, Industrial Statistics Section and the UN Comtrade database.

Figure 5.2 Trends in per capita cigarette consumption, 1971, 1981 and 1991

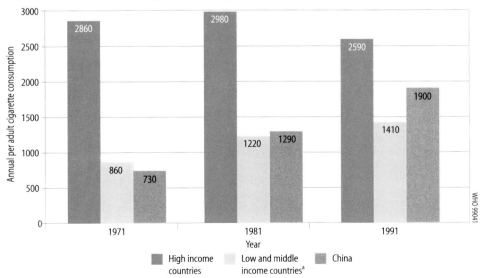

[a]Data for China are also included in low and middle income countries.

Source: *Tobacco or health: A global status report.* Geneva, World Health Organization, 1997.

THE ECONOMIC COSTS

Tobacco obviously provides economic benefits to producers. Similarly, the fact that users are willing to pay for tobacco products means that they clearly derive measurable benefits from them. However, economic analyses conclude that even with highly conservative assumptions, the economic costs of tobacco exceed its estimated benefits (see Box 5.1).

One analysis by Barnum *(7)* tried to estimate the additional costs – in mortality, morbidity and health care – and the benefits – to consumers and producers – per year if global tobacco production were to increase by 1000 metric tons. The analysis concluded that there would be net economic losses of 13.6 million dollars per year, and said: "Tobacco is a poor investment if the objective is to enhance the future welfare of the globe". In fact there has been a 26% increase in production between 1994 and 1997 – equal to almost 2.1 million metric tons, giving a total of just over 8 million metric tons.

The effect of tobacco-related mortality on economic growth can be estimated from the statistical models of the determinants of economic growth discussed in Chapter 1.

Box 5.1 The economics of tobacco control

While health policy-makers accept that smoking should be controlled, there is still widespread debate and uncertainty within governments about the economic consequences of such action. Many policy-makers fear that raising taxes on cigarettes would cut government revenues; that sharply reduced demand for tobacco would mean catastrophic job losses for economies; or that health systems would have to spend more if there were fewer smokers because smokers die young, sparing societies the cost of caring for them in their old age.

The World Bank's study team of economists has examined each of these issues and concludes that the policy-makers' fears are largely unfounded. On the contrary, there are strong grounds for intervening, with minimal costs. For example, even a modest tax increase of 10% would prevent 7 million deaths, including those of people in productive middle age, in low income countries. The team has produced a report[1] whose key recommendations are to increase taxes on manufactured tobacco worldwide, to support specific information so that the addictive nature of nicotine and the damage caused by tobacco are understood by consumers and governments, and to deregulate nicotine replacement therapies.

Since 1991 the World Bank has had a formal policy of not lending for tobacco production and of encouraging tobacco control. The Bank works in close partnership with WHO. The following key messages on the economics of tobacco control provide answers to commonly asked questions.

- **Do not individuals "freely" choose to consume tobacco? Many know the risks. Why, then, should governments discourage smoking?**

Most smokers start when they are children or adolescents – when they have incomplete information about the risks of tobacco and its addictive nature. By the time they try to stop many are addicted. Governments can adopt policies to correct these information and addiction problems. Furthermore, governments are right to restrict smokers from exposing other people to the risks and nuisance of passive smoking.

- **Do the economic costs of tobacco control – for example, unemployment on tobacco farms – substantially outweigh potential health benefits?**

No. There may well be temporary income loss among producers and distributors of tobacco. Successful control policies will lead to only a slow decline in global tobacco use (which is projected to stay high for several decades). The resulting need for downsizing will be far less dramatic than many other industries have had to face. Furthermore, money not spent on tobacco will be spent on other goods, generating alternative employment. Economists have concluded that the economic benefits of tobacco control far exceed the costs.

- **If tobacco addiction is so strong, why would raising taxes produce any health benefits?**

The vast majority of numerous studies have shown that increased taxes lead to fewer smokers and fewer deaths. Price increases deter adolescents more than adults, so they may not become addicted at all. People in developing countries are more price responsive than in high income countries.

- **Won't governments lose revenues if they increase cigarette taxes, because people will buy fewer cigarettes? Raising tobacco taxes will be thwarted by smuggling and illicit production – so, again, why raise taxes?**

Calculations show that very substantial cigarette tax increases will still reduce consumption and increase tax revenues, even in the face of smuggling. The magnitude of smuggling is linked to organized crime, and has also been linked in a number of recent cases to the activities of the tobacco industry itself. Governments can adopt effective policies to control it, such as stopping street sales, and by using warning labels and prominent tax stamps.

- **In many countries, poor people smoke more than do the affluent. Are not cigarette tax increases regressive, that is, they hurt the poor?**

While smoking levels increase with income early in a country's tobacco epidemic, with time the poor and uneducated smoke more than do the affluent. Moreover, the study finds that smoking explains much of the gap in middle-age mortality between rich and poor groups. Cigarette tax increases, even so, need not be regressive. In some cases tax increases have reduced consumption by the poor so much that their smoking expenditures actually declined. More importantly, health benefits from cigarette taxes are highly progressive: greater reductions in tobacco use by poor people and minority groups in response to price increases improve their health.

[1] *Curbing the epidemic: Governments and the economics of tobacco control.* Washington DC, The World Bank, 1999.

OBSTACLES TO TOBACCO CONTROL

Evidence about the addictive nature of nicotine, and other ill-effects of smoking, needs to be disseminated more widely. The tobacco industry is reluctantly surrendering its secrets.

LACK OF INFORMATION ON RISKS

Like consumers of other goods, tobacco consumers need information about what they are buying. Tobacco, however, differs from most consumer goods in that it has harmful health consequences and is addictive. Therefore its consumers have to weigh up an additional type of information in making their decision to buy. The extent to which smokers know about the health consequences and addictive nature of their purchase is critical in determining what they believe they are buying.

Consumers can learn about the health effects of tobacco in several ways. One is through published scientific and epidemiological research which may be summarized in the media. They may also learn through warning labels directly attached to cigarette packs. A third way is through public information campaigns, or counter-advertising; a fourth is through educational initiatives, such as school and community programmes. All of these have been shown to be effective to varying degrees; further research is required on educational initiatives in high income countries in reducing demand for tobacco. A Surgeon General's report in the United States and a Royal College of Physicians report in the United Kingdom, both published in the 1960s, have been responsible for halting much of the increases in consumption in those countries. The implication is that a greater increase in the availability of health information in developing countries would be expected to lead to a significant decrease in global tobacco consumption.

All countries need to increase and improve local studies on tobacco-attributable mortality. Established vital registration systems, some of them over 100 years old, can be used in some rich countries to assess disease patterns and trends. Decades of epidemiological research have identified some of the particular causes of such trends, particularly tobacco use. This is not yet so in poorer countries.

Unfortunately, country-specific information on tobacco-related disease is weakest precisely in the countries where the epidemic looms largest. Recently, WHO collaborating centres and Chinese scientists have helped to develop an innovative model where simply asking about smoking on death certificates provides a low-cost and reliable method of monitoring the tobacco epidemic. Similar methods could be used to monitor the hazards of tobacco in many other populations. For example, in South Africa smoking status is routinely reported on the new type of death certificate, perhaps obviating the need to interview family members.

TOBACCO USE IS AN ADDICTION

As many millions of smokers have belatedly discovered – and lack of information is partly to blame – nicotine is addictive. Some addiction experts have rated tobacco as worse than heroin or cocaine in producing dependency. The 1988 report of the United States Surgeon General, subtitled *Nicotine addiction,* concluded that: "The pharmacological and behavioural processes that determine tobacco addiction are similar to those that determine addiction to drugs such as heroin and cocaine"*(8).*

Tobacco satisfies the criteria for "dependence" in the tenth revision of the International Classification of Diseases *(9).* Classification F17 is entitled *Mental and behavioural disorders due to use of tobacco.* Sub-classification F17.2, *Dependence syndrome,* offers a description that will be familiar to most smokers: a cluster of behavioural, cognitive and physiological phenomena that develop after repeated substance use and that typically include a strong desire to take the drug, difficulties in controlling its use, persisting in use despite harmful consequences, a higher priority given to drug use than to other activities and obligations, increased tolerance, and sometimes a physical withdrawal state.

Research suggests that the process by which people decide about tobacco usage involves a "tobacco addiction cycle". This consists of the stages a person goes through when he or she changes from being a "non-smoker" into a "new smoker", then becomes a "committed smoker", then typically a "smoker trying to stop" and, for a fortunate minority, a "reformed smoker" who, alas, is liable to start the cycle all over again *(6)*.

Many people consume tobacco primarily to obtain nicotine, which is found in all tobacco products. Cigarettes are highly refined vehicles designed to give rapid peak nicotine levels. In the words of the tobacco industry, "Think of the cigarette as a dispenser for a dose unit of nicotine"*(10)*. The nicotine is quickly absorbed via the lungs of smokers and reaches the brain within seconds. It is the primary active ingredient in tobacco that reinforces the biomedical and behavioural process of individual smoking habits. Social and psychological influences are also important in the initiation of smoking, but the addictive nature of nicotine is the main reason why many smokers maintain their tobacco use *(8)*, leading to tobacco-related ill-health, disability and premature death.

Nicotine addiction is not simply a matter of choice or taste. It is not irreversibly addictive, as many people can quit smoking. This explains much of the decline in smoking among adults in OECD countries. But some people find quitting virtually impossible. Even smokers who quit often have to make several attempts before dropping the habit; and former smokers remain vulnerable to resuming smoking at times of stress.

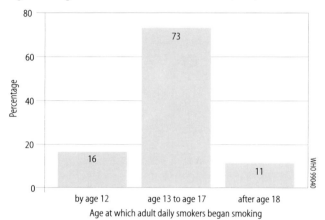

Figure 5.3 Age at which nicotine addiction starts, USA, 1991

Source: **Committee on Preventing Addiction in Children and Youths, Institute of Medicine.**
Growing up tobacco free, preventing nicotine addiction in children and youths. Washington DC,
National Academy Press, 1994.

Nicotine addiction takes hold almost exclusively in children and youth (see Figure 5.3). About half to three-quarters of teenagers in OECD countries try smoking, and about half of those quit quickly. The rest become life-long smokers, among whom one in two will die from smoking. The joint probability of trying smoking, becoming addicted and dying prematurely is higher than for any other addiction (such as alcohol, for which the likelihood of addiction is much lower). Also, children taking up smoking are more likely to experiment with other drugs than those who do not.

Nicotine addiction creates an incentive for the tobacco industry to subsidize or give away free cigarettes to potential smokers, especially young people, in order to induce them to smoke, and otherwise to keep prices high to maximize profits. The same incentive applies to creating addiction among adults in developing countries by manipulating price.

TOBACCO DEALERS MAKE ENORMOUS PROFITS

Tobacco is big business (see Table 5.2). This year, twice as many cigarettes will be smoked as were lit 30 years ago. The tobacco industry is expanding, with the world retail market in cigarettes now worth some US$ 300 billion. Tobacco companies continue to make huge profits, estimated at more than $20 billion a year.

The tobacco industry exerts its influence in countries in several ways: politically as a result of large profits, through denial of tobacco's health impacts, and by advertising and promoting cigarettes. The cigarette market is rapidly expanding among developing countries. Globally, about 6000 billion cigarettes are consumed each year, up from 3000 billion in 1970, despite the fall in countries such as Australia, Canada, Japan, New Zealand, the UK, the USA, and most northern European countries *(11)*. For example, total cigarette consumption in the United Kingdom has fallen from 138 billion to 80 billion per year over the last two decades.

Developing countries are an ideal target for market expansion. In the past few decades, transnational tobacco conglomerates have made tremendous inroads into the markets of poor and middle income nations in Africa, Asia, Eastern Europe and Latin America. Manufacturers have benefited from the globalization of trade, creating big increases in domestic tobacco consumption and imports of tobacco products in many low and middle income nations. In many countries, tobacco companies support social services, in an attempt to portray themselves as purveying "just another product".

Like other industries, the tobacco industry has no financial incentive to provide health information that would reduce consumption of its products. On the contrary, the industry has consistently hidden product information on the ill effects of smoking, used the power of its advertising dollars to dissuade lay journals from reporting on smoking's health effects, and resorted to other methods to decrease information available to smokers. Internal industry documents uncovered in recent American lawsuits confirm such practices *(12)*. Furthermore, the industry has played an active role in funding and disseminating research that casts doubt on the links between tobacco and death. The impact of such information on overall consumer knowledge is difficult to assess. But it is likely to have impeded individual assessments of the true risks of smoking, and it has slowed the spread of government-initiated anti-smoking information campaigns.

Advertising is a crucial component of the industry's expansion. It is the primary method of competition within a highly concentrated industry which has a small number of rela-

Table 5.2 The ten largest tobacco companies, 1997

	Cigarettes (billions)	Cigarette production (% of total)	Tobacco sales (US$ millions)	Leading brand names
1. China National Tobacco Corporation (China)	1 700	24.6	...	Zhong Hua, Hong Ta Shan
2. Philip Morris (United States of America)	947	13.7	23 895	Marlboro, Virginia Slims
3. BAT – British American Tobacco (United Kingdom)[a]	712	10.3	11 845	Derby
4. R.J. Reynolds (United States of America)	316	4.6	8 325	Winston, Camel
5. Japan Tobacco (Japan)	288	4.2	23 445	Mild Seven
6. Rothmans International (South Africa)[a]	187	2.7	5 500	Rothmans
7. Reemtsma (Germany)	119	1.7	2 330	West
8. KT&G – Korea Tobacco and Ginseng Corporation (Republic of Korea)	94	1.4	...	This
9. Tekel (Turkey)	75	1.1	1 550	Maltepe
10. Seita (France)	55	0.8	3 125	Gauloises
Others	2 407	34.9	...	

[a] Merged in 1999.
... Data not available.

Source: *World Tobacco File 1998–2001*, London, International Trade Publications Ltd., 1998.

tively large firms. These firms tend not to compete by price, but try to increase sales with advertising. The largest international tobacco companies are Philip Morris and BAT (see Table 5.2). *Advertising age* reports that in 1996, for advertising outside of the USA, Philip Morris was the ninth largest advertiser in the world and BAT was the 44th largest. In addition, an *Advertising age* survey of Asia, Europe and the Middle East finds that tobacco companies are listed in the top ten advertisers in 21 out of 50 countries.

Huge increases in cigarette advertising and a 10% increase in total tobacco use occurred in four Asian countries when US cigarette companies entered those markets *(13)*. Increases in consumption come both from new consumers and from increased tobacco use by existing consumers. In the case of cigarettes, new consumers are often uninformed adolescents.

PRINCIPLES OF CONTROL

Effective tobacco control policies and interventions can make a real difference to tobacco prevalence and consumption, and hence to associated health outcomes. Most of the documented successes have occurred in industrialized countries, but some developing countries have recently introduced effective measures. Protection of children, protection of non-smokers, informing adult smokers in order to encourage cessation, and improving equity are key objectives. All are served by interventions to reduce the demand for and supply of tobacco products, but to differing degrees. Table 5.3 shows the instruments of tobacco control policies ranked by priority to achieve their goals.

One major cross-national study has analysed the individual and combined effects of a range of policies and interventions on future prevalence *(14)*. Their relevance to countries in varying stages of economic development is summarized in Table 5.4. Price increases (through excise taxes on tobacco products) constitute by far the most important policy tool available. The other interventions have demonstrated effectiveness when properly enacted and enforced. The study highlights the need for policy-makers to use the best mix of policies. These measures are relatively inexpensive, and can more than finance themselves through tobacco taxes. Each can be recommended for inclusion in a typical national tobacco control strategy.

Which combination works best will depend on the particular country and the particular time, although significant taxation levels are likely to figure prominently in most contexts.

CREATING A "FAIR INFORMATION" ENVIRONMENT

This can be achieved by conveying accurate, evidence-based public health information on the risks of tobacco. It also entails a complete, worldwide ban of all tobacco advertising

Table 5.3 Goals and principles of tobacco control policies

Principles	Goals		
	Prevent new addictions	Reduce general consumption	Facilitate cessation
1. Ban advertising and expand public health information	■■	■■■	■■
2. Use taxes and regulations to reduce consumption	■■■	■■■	■■
3. Encourage cessation of tobacco use	■	■■	■■■
4. Build anti-tobacco coalitions	■	■■■	■

■■■ high priority   ■■ medium priority   ■ low priority

Table 5.4 Principles to guide tobacco control policies in different countries

Principles	Low income countries	Countries in transition	Middle income countries	High income countries
Principle 1				
Bans on advertising and promotion	■ ■ ■	■ ■ ■	■ ■ ■	■ ■ ■
Public health information	■ ■	■ ■	■ ■ ■	■ ■
Principle 2				
Increased taxation	■ ■	■ ■ ■	■ ■ ■	■ ■
Regulation to reduce public and workplace smoking	■	■ ■	■ ■ ■	■ ■ ■
Principle 3				
Deregulation of nicotine-replacement products	■	■ ■	■ ■ ■	■ ■ ■
Principle 4				
Anti-tobacco coalitions	■	■ ■	■ ■ ■	■ ■

■ ■ ■ highly relevant   ■ ■ relevant   ■ somewhat relevant

and promotion that convey biased messages and seductive images. Further, it requires full disclosure by the tobacco industry about their practices that affect public policy.

Mass public information and media campaigns involve both mass counter-advertising efforts and large and serious warning labels on tobacco products. Recent evidence from counter-advertising campaigns that are financed by earmarked cigarette taxes *(15)* have shown reductions in smoking. Strong and varied health warnings written in local languages, as have been used in Canada and South Africa, are also needed.

Research on the causes, consequences and costs of tobacco use has contributed to a social climate where effective tobacco control can occur. Priority research is required in the world's major regions to support action on tobacco control, as there is a lack of such information in most low and middle income countries, and governments and health officials may dismiss evidence that is not local or regional.

USING TAXES AND REGULATIONS TO REDUCE CONSUMPTION

Higher tobacco prices result in lower consumption among all age groups, but the young and poor are most affected. Regulations that forbid advertising, promotional distribution, vending machine sales, smoking in public places and under-age smoking complement taxes in reducing consumption. Partial restrictions on advertising may be ineffective – leading to promotion through other media. There is substantial evidence that advertising and promotion target children, who are least informed about the risks of tobacco use.

Regular and sustained tax increases – in many cases to a multiple of current levels – would be the most effective tool of any type to control tobacco use. Tax increases reduce smoking among youth more than among adults, and also help to narrow the behavioural gaps between the poor and rich in smoking *(16)*. Contrary to many claims by the tobacco industry, increasing tax rates reduces consumption and, in the short to medium term, increases government revenue.

China is perhaps the best recent example of the potential health and revenue benefit of appropriate taxation. In China, tobacco taxation has been a major source of revenue for many years. A recent World Bank report on financing health services suggested that a 10% additional tax on tobacco could cut consumption by 5% while generating an additional

4.5% increase in revenue. This extra revenue would cover more than a third of the incremental funds needed for provision of basic health services for China's poorest 100 million inhabitants *(17)*.

ENCOURAGING CESSATION OF TOBACCO USE

This can be achieved in part by encouraging markets for less harmful and less expensive ways of delivering nicotine. Although nicotine is the addictive substance in tobacco, it causes relatively little harm itself. For many current smokers, continued use of nicotine – through patches, tablets, inhalers or other means – offers the best practical approach to cessation.

Under new proposals announced by the UK government in December 1998, £60 million was being made available to set up a comprehensive service within the NHS to help people stop smoking. Proposals included providing a week's supply of nicotine patches free to smokers on low incomes. Deregulation of nicotine replacement products should permit governments to improve the success of tobacco control. Such products are increasingly available in Western countries, but they are much less available in low and middle income countries.

BUILDING TOBACCO CONTROL COALITIONS, DEFUSING OPPOSITION TO CONTROL MEASURES

Public revenues, especially those from tobacco taxes, can fund groups and activities that will advance the movement towards control. They can also selectively fund the short-run transition to other employment for individuals, such as tobacco farmers, whose livelihoods might be affected by reduced consumption. Governments can help to mobilize civil society and other groups by funding the equivalent of a "tobacco or health" unit. Several models for such units exist. They are usually independent of governments, but may have discretion over public finances used to decrease consumption. Such units have existed in Australia and the United States (California and Massachusetts), and have been financed by tobacco taxes. The benefits of earmarking are to help concentrate potential "winners" such as other health groups, behind tobacco control.

For example, the Victoria Health Promotion Foundation (VicHealth) in Australia was established in 1987 and funded until 1997 through a small percentage tax on tobacco products. It sponsors sports and arts events that the tobacco industry has traditionally found attractive. Now, instead of these events being used to recruit smokers, VicHealth promotes the benefits of not smoking and of adopting a healthy lifestyle. It also supports other health promotion programmes in areas such as injury prevention, healthy eating and physical activity. The gains for the community are considerable, and the lives of millions of Victorians have been enriched and enlivened by participating in VicHealth funded programmes.

Tobacco control coalitions have gained invaluable ammunition by taking the industry to court and forcing the disclosure of its documents. In the United States in 1998, the State of Minnesota and medical insurance groups successfully sued the industry for consumer fraud, winning not just US$ 7 billion, but the disclosure of almost four million of the industry's internal documents, totalling about 35 million pages, dating back to the 1950s. The documents, now stored in a depository in Minneapolis, Minnesota and open to public inspection, relate to the medical evidence on smoking, the addictiveness of nicotine, and marketing strategies, among other subjects. This information may have a huge impact on tobacco litigation and campaigns for comprehensive tobacco control measures in other countries. Other States, such as South Carolina, have similarly obtained previously hidden documents.

TOBACCO CONTROL:
WHAT SOME COUNTRIES HAVE ACHIEVED

The chief goal of tobacco control policies is to reduce damage to societies from smoking. Such policies offer enormous health benefits, and have been successful in many developed countries. A World Bank report (see Box 5.1) suggests that with a worldwide price increase in cigarettes of only 10%, 40 million people will quit smoking (representing 3% of all smokers in 1995) and eventually almost 20 million deaths attributable to smoking will be averted. Such an increase would also result in a decrease in consumption of 384 billion cigarettes per year *(6)*. Some countries have already shown the way, and their achievements can be models for others (see Box 5.2).

Thailand has adopted a comprehensive control programme. Smoking in cinemas and buses was banned in Bangkok in the 1970s. National advertising bans and other anti-smoking measures followed and in 1993 the government raised cigarette tax on health grounds. In 1997, it became the first country after Canada to require tobacco companies to reveal the ingredients of their cigarettes. Overall smoking prevalence has dropped by 4% among males and by almost 3% among 15–19-year-olds.

The United Kingdom has reduced smoking substantially, through both price and non-price measures. From 1965 to 1995 annual UK cigarette sales fell from 150 billion to 80

Box 5.2 Towards a tobacco-free Europe

Over 30% of adults in the European Region are regular daily smokers. It is estimated that one in five of all 35-year-old men in the eastern part of the Region will die from the effects of smoking before they reach the age of 70. This is twice as high as in western Europe. Non-smokers are at risk, too, of disease resulting from breathing other people's smoke. Smoking is currently on the increase, predominantly in the central and eastern countries of the Region, and women and children are particularly targeted by the tobacco industries. The behaviour of some adolescent smokers is shown in the table.

There are no economic benefits from tobacco, as global costs outweigh the profits. A proportion of tobacco taxes is sufficient to fund all tobacco control activities, including support to sports and artistic events that were sponsored by the tobacco industry until the European Parliament decided in July 1998 to ban advertising and sponsorship by tobacco companies.

Because of the time lag between smoking and death from smoking-related causes, the main determinant of the level of tobacco-related deaths over the next 35 years in the European Region will be the number of the existing 180 million smokers who can successfully quit the habit or at least significantly reduce their consumption. In the USA, recognition of the addictive nature of nicotine led the Food and Drug Administration to acquire jurisdiction over cigarettes. This move needs to be replicated in other countries, as deciding who controls the delivery of nicotine and how it is regulated will determine the number of deaths caused by tobacco in the future.

Most smokers concede that public places should be smoke-free, and most of them wish to stop smoking. Cessation advice and interventions are highly cost-effective. The cost per life year gained is below US$3000 in Western European countries for counselling for smoking cessation, with or without nicotine replacement therapy, compared with $23 000 for blood pressure screening of 40-year-old men and a median cost of $30 000 for over 300 standard medical interventions. There is no doubt that effective, coordinated action has an impact. In France, cigarette consumption has declined considerably since the Evin law of 1991 banned tobacco advertising, restricted smoking in public places and introduced price increases.

Percentage of 15-year-old boys and girls smoking at least once a week, selected European countries, 1989–1990 and 1993–1994

	Boys		Girls	
	1989–1990	1993–1994	1989–1990	1993–1994
Austria	23	29	20	31
Finland	33	30	32	26
France (Nancy and Toulouse)	...	23	...	25
Hungary	31	25	20	19
Poland	20	23	10	13
Russian Federation (St Petersburg)	...	19	...	10
Spain	18	20	27	27
Sweden	15	15	20	19
UK - Northern Ireland	...	23	...	25
UK - Scotland	16	21	18	26
UK - Wales	14	18	22	27

... Data not available.

Source: *Smoking, drinking and drug taking in the European Region.* Copenhagen, WHO Regional Office for Europe, 1997.

Contributed by the WHO Regional Office for Europe.

billion. Annual UK tobacco deaths in the 35–69 year age group decreased from 80 000 to 40 000. In December 1998, the UK government announced a major campaign to help 1.5 million people to stop smoking by the year 2010; it said taxes on tobacco products would continue to be increased. The government's targets by the year 2010 include reducing smoking among children in England from 13% to 9%, reducing adult smoking from 28% to 24% or less, and reducing the number of women who smoke during pregnancy from 23% to 15%.

The European Union has a multi-pronged approach to tobacco control. An EU Directive on tobacco advertising became law in June 1998. All EU Member States are now required to introduce legislation to implement the directive, which calls for bans on direct and indirect sponsorship leading to a complete ban by 1 October 2006. This means that there should be a ban on advertising and promotion, except in print media, within 3 years; a ban on advertising in print media within 4 years; a ban on tobacco sponsorship of all events not organized at the world level within 5 years; and, no later than 1 October 2006, a ban on sponsorship of events organized at the world level (for example, Formula 1 motor racing) on a case by case basis, subject to voluntary worldwide controls and declining tobacco funding. Member States of the EU may introduce tougher or additional measures and more rapid implementation timetables than required by the directive.

France has had a comprehensive tobacco control law fully in force since 1993. The law bans tobacco advertising and requires strong health warnings on both the front and the back of the package. It also controls smoking in transport, public places and workplaces by either banning it altogether or limiting it to just a few smoking areas. Between 1991, when the law was adopted, and 1995, tobacco consumption, measured in weight of tobacco products sold, had fallen by 7.3%.

The United States had health education campaigns combined with smoke-free policies between 1965 and 1985 that resulted in 40 million people not starting to smoke, or giving up the habit. There were about 50 million smokers in the United States in 1985, but there would have been 90 million without the measures that were introduced. The difference represents many hundreds of thousands of lives saved.

Among Latin American countries, advertising controls apply in Chile, Colombia, Costa Rica, Mexico and Panama. Smoking is banned in domestic and international flights throughout the Americas. National tobacco control plans have been drafted in Brazil and Mexico.

Norway enforced a total ban on all tobacco advertising in 1975, imposed health warnings and prohibited the sales of cigarettes to minors. The legislation had a huge impact on tobacco sales, especially among young teenagers. It is estimated that if consumption in general had continued rising it would be about 80% higher than it actually is.

WHO's Tobacco Free Initiative

The deadly impact of tobacco on health now and in the future is the primary reason for WHO's strong explicit support to tobacco control on a worldwide basis. WHO established the Tobacco Free Initiative in July 1998 to coordinate an improved global strategic response.

The long-term mission of global tobacco control is to reduce smoking prevalence and tobacco consumption in all countries and among all groups, and thereby reduce the burden of disease caused by tobacco.

In support of this mission, the goals of the Tobacco Free Initiative are to:
- galvanize global support for evidence-based tobacco control policies and actions;
- build new partnerships for action and strengthen existing ones;

- heighten awareness of the need to address tobacco issues at all levels of society;
- accelerate the implementation of national, regional and global strategies;
- commission policy research to support rapid, sustained and innovative actions;
- mobilize resources to support required actions.

To achieve these goals, the Tobacco Free Initiative will build strong external partnerships with a range of organizations and institutions around the world and internally throughout WHO headquarters and its regional and country offices (see Box 5.3). Success will be measured in terms of actions at local, country and global levels that achieve better tobacco control.

The Tobacco Free Initiative will take a global leadership role in promoting effective policies and interventions that make a real difference to tobacco prevalence and associated health outcomes. Evidence shows that countries which undertake concerted and comprehensive actions to address tobacco control can bring about significant reductions in tobacco-related harm. It is important to consider the best mix of specific interventions required. In a broad policy framework, the mix will vary according to each country's political, social, cultural and economic reality. Actions that could be included in a comprehensive national tobacco control policy are shown in Table 5.4.

The Tobacco Free Initiative will launch WHO's "World No-Tobacco Day" in 1999 (an annual event celebrated on 31 May) with the slogan "Leaving the pack behind", putting the emphasis on cessation. This event and related activities are aimed at building awareness of

---

Box 5.3 Activities of the Tobacco Free Initiative

The Tobacco Free Initiative is building on WHO's collaboration with the following partners in order to extend opportunities for tobacco control.

- UNICEF: to prevent children and adolescents from starting to smoke.
- World Bank: to use excise taxes effectively; to dispell myths about financial benefits.
- US Centers for Disease Control and Prevention (CDC): to support global surveillance of tobacco use and its consequences.
- Environmental Protection Agency (EPA): to reach environmental constituencies.
- US National Institutes of Health (NIH); International Development and Research Centre (IDRC), Canada; Swedish International Development Authority (SIDA): to expand the evidence base through policy research.
- International nongovernmental organizations: to strengthen ac-

tion at grass-roots level; to promote networking through the Internet.
- Private sector: to channel energy and expertise from pharmaceutical, media and entertainment industries into tobacco control activities.
- Academic centres: to build capacity in several disciplines; to stimulate research for action.

The Tobacco Free Initiative is developing a Framework Convention on Tobacco Control, which was initiated by WHO's Member States at the World Health Assembly in May 1996. The aim is for Member States to adopt the convention and key protocol agreements at the Health Assembly no later than May 2003. In May 1999, they will consider the next steps to be taken in the negotiation process.

The WHO Framework Convention on Tobacco Control represents the first time that the Organization has exercised its constitutional mandate under Article 19 to encourage nations to develop a convention. If a convention is

adopted and enters into force, it will be the first time that a convention approach has been specifically applied to address a global public health problem.

WHO will build consensus, mobilize support, and encourage adoption of the WHO Framework Convention and related protocols. The analytical work will focus on global and national law, trade issues, political mapping, and industry analysis and monitoring. A two-year cycle of continuous and enhanced international legal support, involving experts from industrialized and developing countries as well as international lawyers with extensive experience with the negotiation of international treaties, has been initiated.

A technical consultation of public health experts was held in Canada in December 1998. This meeting provided recommendations regarding the role of the Organization in promoting the WHO Framework Convention; possible elements of the Convention; special support to developing coun-

tries; and means of advancing adoption of the Convention. To ensure the active participation of developing countries in the negotiation of the WHO Framework Convention, another technical consultation will be held in India in 1999. This meeting will involve participants from various government ministries, nongovernmental organizations, and other international organizations and will focus on developing country issues that should be addressed in formulating and implementing the Convention. It is expected that this meeting will provide a foundation for country-specific consultations, with a view to establishing "model" national committees to support the convention process.

The role of the WHO Secretariat in the treaty-making process is to provide technical support and guidance to Member States in the pre-negotiation and negotiation phases.

the health hazards of smoking and fostering behaviour change supportive of cessation among the general public, health professionals and United Nations agency staff. It will involve partnerships with nongovernmental organizations and the private sector, including the pharmaceutical industry.

In 1996, WHO's Member States initiated the development of a Framework Convention on Tobacco Control. A framework convention is a form of treaty which is an international instrument between States, or between States and international organizations, governed by international law. The approach being proposed consists of two parts: a framework convention that calls for cooperation in achieving broadly stated goals and establishes the general norms and institutions of a multilateral legal structure; and protocols which elaborate additional or more specific commitments and institutional arrangements designed to implement these goals. The groundwork has been completed and the process of developing and negotiating the framework convention has been accelerated (see Box 5.3). The objectives are to establish an intergovernmental negotiating committee by 2000, and the adoption of the convention and key protocol agreements by 2003.

Although the drafting and negotiation of conventions is a prerogative of States, experience has demonstrated that international and nongovernmental organizations can actively facilitate the treaty-making process. Backed by the prominence of an internationally accepted legal instrument, global action can move ahead more effectively. By employing the policies and measures described in this chapter, governments are better-equipped than ever before to combat the tobacco epidemic and reduce its appalling toll.

REFERENCES

1. **Peto R et al.** *Mortality from smoking in developed countries 1950–2000.* New York, Oxford University Press, 1994.

2. **Parkin DM et al.** At least one in seven cases of cancer is caused by smoking. Global estimates for 1985. *International journal of cancer*, 1994, **59**(4): 494–504.

3. *The world health report 1997 – Conquering suffering, enriching humanity.* Geneva, World Health Organization, 1997.

4. *Curbing the epidemic: Governments and the economics of tobacco control.* Washington, The World Bank, 1999.

5. *World development report 1993 – Investing in health.* New York, Oxford University Press for The World Bank, 1993.

6. **Murray CJL, Lopez AD.** *The global burden of disease.* Cambridge MA, Harvard University Press, 1996.

7. **Barnum H.** *Initial analysis of the economic costs and benefits of investing in tobacco.* Washington, The World Bank, 1993 (unpublished manuscript, Human Development Department).

8. **US Department of Health and Human Services.** *The health consequences of smoking: Nicotine addiction. A report of the Surgeon General.* Rockville MD, Centers for Disease Control, 1988 (DHHS Publication No.CDC 88-8406).

9. *The ICD-10 classification of mental and behavioural disorders. Clinical descriptions and diagnostic guidelines.* Geneva, World Health Organization, 1992.

10. **Dunn WL Jnr.** *Motives and incentives in cigarette smoking.* Philip Morris 1972. Minnesota Tobacco Trial - Exhibit 18089.

11. **Jha P, Chaloupka FJ** (eds). *Tobacco control policies in developing countries.* New York, Oxford University Press, 1999.

12. **Hurt RD, Robertson CR.** Prying open the door to the tobacco industry's secrets about nicotine: The Minnesota tobacco trial. *Journal of the American Medical Association*, 1998, **280**: 1178–1181.

13. **Chaloupka FJ, Laixuthai A.** *US trade policy and cigarette smoking in Asia.* Cambridge MA, National Bureau of Economic Research, 1996 (NBER Working Paper 5543).

14. **Townsend J.** *Tobacco price and the smoking epidemic.* Copenhagen, WHO Regional Office for Europe, 1988 (unpublished document, Smoke-free Europe Series, No. 9).

15. **Hu TW, Sung HY, Keeler TE.** Reducing cigarette consumption in California: Tobacco taxes vs an anti-smoking media campaign. *American journal of public health*, 1995, **85**(9): 1218–1222.

16. **Farrelly MC, Bray JW.** Response to increases in cigarette prices by race/ethnicity, income, and age groups – United States, 1976–1993. *Journal of the American Medical Association*, 1998, **280**(23): 1979–1980.

17. **Saxenian H, McGreevey W.** *China – Issues and options in health financing.* Washington DC, The World Bank, 1996 (Report No.15278).

6

MAKING A DIFFERENCE

A century of remarkable progress has revolutionized the health conditions of most of humanity. Among high income countries, life expectancy increased by 30 to 40 years in this period. Most of today's low and middle income countries have experienced even more dramatic gains, gains that have transformed quality of life and contributed to economic growth.

Yet, as this report has documented, over a billion people will enter the 21st century without having shared in these gains: their lives remain short and scarred by disease. Many others fail to realize their full potential for better health because health systems allocate resources to interventions of low quality or of low efficacy related to cost. Increasing numbers of people forego or defer essential care or suffer huge financial burdens resulting from an unexpected need for expensive services. The continuing challenges to health ministries and to countries thus remain enormous. Meeting those challenges will make a major difference in the quality of life worldwide. And the difference for the poor will not only be in improving their quality of life, but also, through increasing their productivity, in addressing one of the root causes of poverty.

Global leadership and advocacy for health remain critical missing ingredients in the formula for progress. The heart of both Roll Back Malaria and the Tobacco Free Initiative is global leadership. Advocacy, a function of leadership, is required to convey evidence to prime ministers and finance ministers on how investments in the health of the poor can enhance growth and reduce poverty.

With successful leadership the world could end the first decade of the 21st century with notable accomplishments. Most of the world's poor would no longer suffer today's burden of premature death and excessive disability, and poverty itself would be much reduced. Healthy life expectancy would increase for all. Smoking and other risks to health would fade in significance. The financial risks of unexpected medical needs would be more fairly shared, leaving no household exposed to economic ruin as a result of health expenditure. And health systems would respond with greater compassion, quality and efficiency to the increasingly diverse demands they face. Progress in the 20th century points to the feasibility of reaching these goals. Compressing the time required to accomplish these results is the challenge to leadership in the 21st century.

The potential is there. This report has argued that the tools exist, despite the scale of the challenges before us, to achieve great progress within the first decade of the coming century. What, specifically, are the main challenges?

- First and foremost, *there is a need to reduce greatly the burden of excess mortality and morbidity suffered by the poor.* The OECD's Development Assistance Committee has established the target of halving the number of people living in absolute poverty by the year 2015. This goal is attainable but it will require major shifts in the way that governments all over the world use their resources. It will mean focusing more on interventions that can achieve the greatest health gain possible within prevailing resource limits. It will mean giving renewed attention to diseases like tuberculosis, which disproportionately affect poor people, as well as malaria and HIV/AIDS, which are major constraints to economic growth.

  Women and children suffer poverty more than men; there is therefore a need for greater investments in reducing maternal mortality – and finding ways of improving maternal and childhood nutrition. Reducing the burden of excess mortality and morbidity also means revitalizing and extending the coverage of immunization programmes – still one of the most powerful and cost-effective technologies available. The eradication of poliomyelitis in the Americas in the past decade, and great progress in control elsewhere, hold out the promise that poliomyelitis will join smallpox as a disease known only to history.

- Second, *health systems must proactively counter potential threats to health* resulting from economic crises, unhealthy environments or risky behaviour. Tobacco addiction is perhaps the single most important of these threats. A global commitment to tobacco control – the goal of the Tobacco Free Initiative – can potentially avert scores of millions of premature deaths in the next half century, and its success can point the way for effective control of other threats. Preparing effective responses to emerging infections and countering the spread of resistance to antimicrobials will help insure against the prospect of a significantly increased infectious disease threat. Beyond countering specific threats, promotion of healthy lifestyles underpins a proactive strategy for risk reduction: cleaner air and water, adequate sanitation, healthy diets and safer transportation – all are important. And all are facilitated by stable economic growth and by ensuring that females as well as males have opportunities to increase their educational attainment.

- Third, *there is a need to develop more effective health systems.* In many parts of the world, health systems are ill-equipped to cope with present demands, let alone those they will face in the future. The institutional problems which limit health sector performance are often common to all public services in a country. But despite their importance, they have been relatively neglected by governments and development agencies alike. Dealing with issues such as pay and incentives in the public sector, priority setting and rationing, and unregulated growth in the private sector constitute some of the most challenging items on the international health agenda.

  Limits exist on what governments can finance and on their capacity to deliver services. Hence the need for public policies that recognize these limits. Governments should retain responsibility for setting broad policy directions, for creating an appropriate regulatory environment, and for finance. At the same time they should seek both to diversify the sources of service provision and to select interventions that, for the resources each country chooses to commit, will provide the maximum gains in health levels and their most equitable distribution.

- Finally, *there is a need to invest in expanding the knowledge base* that made the 20th century revolution in health possible, and that will provide the tools for continued gains in the 21st century. Governments of high income countries and large, research-oriented pharmaceutical companies now invest – and will continue to invest – massive resources in research and development oriented to the needs of the more affluent. Much of this investment benefits all humanity, but at least two critical gaps remain. One concerns research and development relevant to the infectious diseases that overwhelmingly afflict the poor. The other concerns the systematic generation of an information base that countries can use in shaping the future of their own health systems.

These challenges provide a sense of direction – for national governments, for members of the international community and for WHO as well. Each of these diverse actors will have its own specific needs, values and capacities; and each may find some of the challenges of little relevance to its own circumstances. What is important for each, however, is to focus its resources where they can make a difference.

The financial resources for health lie overwhelmingly *within* countries. Responsibility for success (or failure) thus lies ultimately with governments. Only a tiny fraction of resources for health in low and middle income countries originates in the international system – development banks, bilateral development assistance agencies, international nongovernmental organizations, foundations and WHO. Health spending in low and middle income countries in 1994 totalled about $250 billion, of which only $2 or 3 billion was from development assistance *(1,2)*. For WHO to make a difference it must therefore focus its country work where the health gains will be highest. Two general guidelines will assist in achieving that focus.

First, concentrating technical assistance on countries with a shared strategic vision will enhance impact. Outsiders should avoid imposing their own perspectives but, rather, support projects and policies to which governments are committed. Concentrating resources on poor countries or vulnerable groups without alternative sources of finance will also amplify impact. A World Bank review of what works in development assistance – and of what fails – found strong support for these principles *(3)*. When development assistance was used to support governments with sound policies it contributed significantly to economic growth and poverty reduction, particularly in poorer countries. But when external actors pushed against the grain of weak national policies they failed. The World Bank further concluded that far too much development assistance has indeed been wasted for just this reason. If WHO is to make a difference the implication is clear: concentrate country-specific technical assistance for health on countries whose policies reflect a shared vision of reaching the poor and of efficiency in health system development.

Second, the international community should avoid using its resources for what individual countries can do for themselves. International resources should, instead, concentrate on functions where international collective action is required *(4)*. These tasks include:
- global leadership and advocacy for health;
- generating and disseminating an evidence and information base for all countries to use;
- catalyzing effective global disease surveillance (as is currently done with influenza, to take an important example);
- setting norms and standards;
- targeting specific global or regional health problems where the concerted action of countries is required (for example, eradication of poliomyelitis);

- helping to provide a voice for those whose health is neglected within their own country or who are stateless;
- ensuring that critical research and development for the poor receives finance.

Making a difference for countries entails – for WHO as for others – focusing the agenda on where the return is highest. This will sometimes be country-specific technical assistance but, more often, working *with* countries on an agenda of common interest will make a greater difference.

REFERENCES

1. *Sector strategy: Health, nutrition and population.* Washington DC, The World Bank, 1997: 4.

2. *Investing in health research and development. Report of the Ad Hoc Committee on Health Research Relating to Future Intervention Options.* Geneva, World Health Organization, 1996 (document TDR/Gen/96.1): 230–231.

3. *Assessing aid.* New York: Oxford University Press for The World Bank, 1998.

4. *Rx for global health cooperation beyond 2000. Report on the Conference on World Health Cooperation Beyond 2000, Mexico City, 29 March–1 April 1998.* Washington DC, Overseas Development Council, 1998.

PART THREE

STATISTICAL ANNEX

For centuries governments have compiled data – for tax and other administrative purposes – concerning characteristics of their populations. With time the potential for comprehensiveness and accuracy has increased and, concomitantly, disparities have grown across countries in data adequacy. All countries maintain at least minimal compilations concerning their economies and their populations; and most countries prepare and distribute these data in categories that share major features with those in other countries. This allows the country's decision-makers to compare characteristics of their own country – or its health system – with other countries (or with their own prior experience).

To achieve maximum benefit from major country investments in generating statistics there needs to be a central service to enhance data comparability and quality, to generate and publish comprehensive sets of data over time, and to identify important common themes. Such an effort must, obviously, deal with the problem of variation in data quality and timeliness; and, in the short term, it must make the best possible use of available data. Over a longer period it is important to encourage and assist countries to improve the quality and scope of their statistical system. WHO is now, through its Global Programme on Evidence for Health Policy, investing substantially in enhancing its capacity to improve demographic and health data, and data systems.

A major initial effort of this Programme involved preparation of estimates of numbers of deaths and disease burden by cause for 1998, and the results of that effort are published for the first time in this Annex. Other tables in the Annex summarize data from WHO programmes, from other agencies and from background research for this report.

EXPLANATORY NOTES

The Statistical Annex includes tables that provide basic data on all Member States and summarize demographic characteristics by WHO Regions (Annex Tables 1 and 5), tables that provide assessments of numbers of deaths and disease burden for some hundred causes by WHO Region (Annex Tables 2–4), tables that characterize the performance of countries on selected aspects of health (Annex Tables 6 and 7), and tables with specific data on incidence, mortality and burden of malaria, tobacco and tuberculosis, which are discussed at some length in the text (Annex Tables 8–10). This highly selective data compilation thus provides a broad overview of global health, economic and health system characteristics and specific information supportive of the main arguments of *The World Health Report.*

The Annex Tables present selected data for individual countries, for countries aggregated by WHO Region and for all Member States combined. The map below delineates the coverage of each of the six WHO Regions, which are: Africa (AFR),

the Americas (AMR), Eastern Mediterranean (EMR), Europe (EUR), South-East Asia (SEAR) and Western Pacific (WPR). Annex Table 1 lists the Member States in each Region alphabetically. Annex Table 5 provides summary demographic data for each Region. The classification of countries into high income, and low and middle income is based on *World development indicators 1998,* Washington DC, The World Bank, 1998. The sums of entries in the Annex Tables may not always equal the totals because of rounding. In some cases, transformations, aggregations and analyses of basic data provide numbers that are more useful to policy-makers than the initial data. Several of the Annex Tables report such transformations, while others report numbers closer to the original categories.

These explanatory notes describe the sources of data and the methods used to calculate the results that the tables report, for each table in turn. Because of their common origin, a single section provides the background for Annex Tables 2–4.

WHO Regional Offices and the areas they serve, 1999

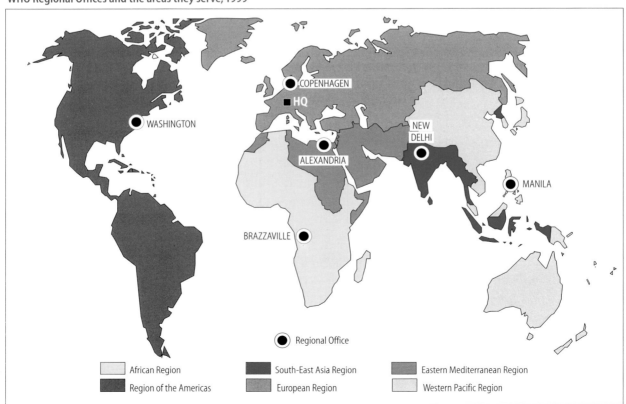

ANNEX TABLE 1

Sources of data and explanation of column headings

Population

1. Total population size in thousands, for 1998. Source: United Nations dataset *World population prospects 1950—2050 (the 1998 revision),* New York, United Nations Population Division, 1998.

2. Annual growth rate has been calculated as the average percentage change in population size between 1978 and 1998. Estimates of population size for 1978 and 1998 were from the United Nations dataset *World population prospects 1950—2020 (the 1998 revision),* New York, United Nations Population Division, 1998.

3. Dependency ratio is defined as the population aged 0–14 and over 65 years as a percentage of the population aged 15–64 years. Estimates of population size for 1978 and 1998 were from the United Nations dataset *World population prospects 1950—2020 (the 1998 revision),* New York, United Nations Population Division, 1998.

4. Total fertility rate is calculated as the average number of children born to a woman of reproductive age. Estimates for 1978 and 1998 were obtained from *World population prospects: The 1998 revision,* New York, United Nations, 1999.

Mortality rates

5. Infant mortality rate (IMR) is defined as the number of deaths per 1000 live births between birth and exact age one year. Estimates are shown for 1978 and 1998. Source: *World population prospects: The 1998 revision,* New York, United Nations, 1999.

6. The probability of dying between birth and exact age 5 years per 1000 live births is shown for male and female children for 1998. Source: Supplementary tabulations to *World population prospects: The 1998 revision* (New York, United Nations, 1999), Population Division, Department of Economic and Social Affairs of the United Nations Secretariat.

7. The probability of dying between age 15 and 59 years per 1000 population, for males and females in that age group, in 1998. Source: Supplementary tabulations to *World population prospects: The 1998 revision* (New York, United Nations, 1999), Population Division, Department of Economic and Social Affairs of the United Nations Secretariat.

8. Maternal mortality ratio (MMR) is defined as the number of maternal deaths per 100 000 live births. The MMR measures the risk of death once a woman has become pregnant. The estimates of MMR for 1990 should be used with caution. Global best estimates for the year 1995 are currently under development. Further information is available from Director, Department of Reproductive Health and Research, WHO, Geneva.

Social and economic

9. Estimates of life expectancy at birth for males and females in 1978 and 1998 were taken from *World population prospects: The 1998 revision,* New York, United Nations, 1999.

10. Real gross domestic product (GDP) per capita adjusted for purchasing power parity is expressed in 1985 US dollars. Data are from the Penn World Table dataset, Mark 5.6, the Chain index, available at: http://www.nber.org/pwt56.html (Summers R, Heston A. The Penn World Table (Mark 5): An expanded set of international comparisons, 1950–1988. *Quarterly journal of economics,* 1991, **106:** 327–368). The annual average growth rate (calculated as the growth rate over a time period divided by the number of years in that period) of GDP per capita is shown for two periods: 1962–1992 and 1982–1992.

11. Educational attainment: the average number of years of education is given for females aged 25 years and above. The inequality in educational attainment between males and females is expressed as the difference in average number of years of education for men and women, aged 25 years or above. Source: Barro R, Lee JW. International measures of schooling years and schooling quality. *American economic review, Papers and proceedings,* 1986, **2:** 218–223.

12. The measure of malnutrition has been chosen to be the percentage of children under age 5 years who are stunted. Stunting is defined as height for age below 2 standard deviations from the international reference median value. Estimates are shown for male and female children for the latest year for which data were available since 1990. Estimates were provided by the Department of Nutrition for Health and Development, Sustainable Development and Healthy Environments Cluster, WHO, Geneva. Regional averages for the period 1975–1995, for both sexes combined can be found in: *WHO global database on child growth and malnutrition* (document WHO/NUT/97.4. Geneva, World Health Organization, 1997). Detailed information on national data disaggregated by sex, age group, urban/rural and regions can be found at: http://www.who.int/whosis/ under *WHO global database on child growth and malnutrition.*

Health services and finance

13. Estimates of the percentage of children immunized against measles are shown for 1987 and 1997. Source: Department of Vaccines and Other Biologicals, Health Technology and Pharmaceuticals Cluster, WHO, Geneva.

14. Data on total health expenditures as a percentage of GDP and the percentage of health expenditures from public sources are taken from: Bos E et al. *Health, nutrition and population indicators: A statistical handbook,* Washington DC, The World Bank, 1999 (Health, nutrition and population series).

ANNEX TABLES 2–4

Methods

We used the following procedures to produce projections for country-level death rates. We began by replicating the original analysis in the 1990 Global Burden of Disease Study (Murray CJL, Lopez AD (eds). *The Global burden of disease: A comprehensive assessment of mortality and disability from diseases, injuries, and risk factors in 1990 and projected to 2020.* Cambridge, Harvard School of Public Health on behalf of the World Health Organization and The World Bank, 1996, Global Burden of Disease and Injury Series, Vol.I), correcting for a number of data and coding errors. This original analysis included explanatory variables (measuring smoking, the logarithm of GDP per capita and its square, the logarithm of human capital, and a time trend serving as a proxy for technology) in a linear regression on logged death rates, with an intercept correction and with missing data deleted listwise. We sought to improve these projections in a number of ways, and evaluated our success in the first instance by calibrating the model with data from 1955 to 1994 and then comparing the forecasts with the actual death rates in 1995. We also tried dropping other years, or multiple years. For all our models, we used multiple imputation (Rubin D. *Multiple imputation for nonresponse in surveys.* New York, Wiley, 1987) via the EMis algorithm (King G et al. Listwise deletion is evil: What to do about missing data in political science? Presented at the annual meeting of the American Political Science Association, Boston, 1998) and *Amelia* software (Honaker J et al. 1999, available for free download at: http://gking.harvard.edu) to cope with the substantial missing data problems.

We used all available variables, along with several lagged variables to make the imputations. This procedure consistently improved the forecasts and so all estimates rely on it. We then tried a long list of candidate models, including various versions of error correction, local trends, partial adjustment, partial pooling via empirical Bayes, fixed effects, and other models. The best model, as judged only by our method of evaluation described above, was one that included no dynamics, used no explanatory variables except technology (i.e. the linear trend term), and included an intercept correction. For example, error correction models did not help despite evidence of nonstationarity, and models with dynamics did not help despite some evidence of time series dependence. Our preference was to use a weighted average of this "best" model and one that included dynamics, but specialists in WHO felt that combining such models produced unreasonable forecasts. We therefore settled on a weighted average of this "best" model and the original 1990 global burden of disease model (with missing data multiply imputed), and with weights elicited from specialists for each cause-of-death disease category. Since there is good reason to think that models that appropriately include dynamics will outperform these forecasts, much work remains to be done.

The final model produced forecasts for the following 16 causes of death and cause-of-death clusters: liver cancer, breast cancer, mouth cancer, stomach cancer, cervix cancer, other cancers, infectious diseases other than HIV/AIDS, tuberculosis and malaria, cardiovascular diseases, respiratory diseases, digestive diseases, all other diseases, road traffic accidents, unintentional injuries, suicide, homicide and violence, and war. We have assumed that the composition of detailed causes within each cause cluster described here for 1998 would be the same as that described in the 1990 global burden of disease analysis. Estimates for HIV/AIDS, lung cancer, malaria and tuberculosis were not based on this model.

Estimates for specific diseases were derived using other methods

1. Tuberculosis. Estimates shown in Annex Tables 2–4 refer to tuberculosis in individuals who are HIV negative. The estimated mortality in individuals infected with tuberculosis who were HIV negative in 1998 was 1.49 million, with a range of 1.1 to 2.2 million deaths. Annex Table 10 provides sex-specific estimates of incidence, deaths and DALYs for HIV-positive and HIV-negative individuals with tuberculosis. For the methods and the source of these estimates see the explanatory note to Annex Table 10.

2. HIV/AIDS. The statistical methods used to estimate AIDS mortality are based in part on the imputation of missing prevalence data from sentinel sites. Further validation of the imputation results would improve the reliability of the method. Furthermore, the application of the gamma distribution to estimate the epidemic curve for the HIV/AIDS epidemic is problematic once the epidemic is established. The estimated trajectory of the epidemic in different countries based on statistical models should be compared with other epidemiological evidence to ensure that the estimates adequately reflect national experience. The estimates of AIDS mortality in sub-Saharan Africa have used national mortality statistics in order to adjust model-based figures. The results will obviously depend on the extent to which these data are reliable, especially with regard to adult mortality levels. UNAIDS and WHO will actively collaborate in further refining and developing these and other methods for reducing the uncertainty in epidemiological estimates of HIV/AIDS within the framework of the UNAIDS/WHO Working Group on Global HIV/AIDS/STD Surveillance.

   For sub-Saharan Africa, the estimated number of deaths from HIV/AIDS in 1998 was 1.83 million with a 95% confidence interval of 1.1 to 2.4 million deaths.

3. Poliomyelitis and Diphtheria. Numbers are rounded to the nearest thousand. Poliomyelitis has been eradicated from the Americas. Apart from that, some deaths occur in all Regions for both conditions.

4. Tetanus. Includes neonatal tetanus (around 300 000 deaths) and tetanus at other ages.

5. Meningitis. Bacterial meningitis and meningococcaemia.

6. Malaria. In Africa, the range for deaths from malaria is estimated to be 758 000 to 1.3 million. The methods used to derive these estimates are described in Annex Table 8.

7. Leprosy. Because of rounding, regional totals exclude an estimated 200 deaths in AFR and AMR, and 100 in EMR and WPR. The total for SEAR is 1400.

8. Maternal conditions. Because of the difficulties inherent in measuring maternal mortality, there is considerable uncertainty around these estimates. The estimated range of maternal deaths in 1998 is 376 to 646 thousand globally. Differences in figures quoted are largely a result of uncertainties about the indirect causes of maternal deaths, estimated to account for 10–20% of maternal mortality. Indirect causes include those resulting from pre-existing disease that developed during pregnancy and was aggravated by the physiological effects of pregnancy, such as malaria, tuberculosis, HIV/AIDS and cardiovascular diseases.

9. Rheumatic heart disease. Does not include other rheumatic diseases.

10. Diabetes. Diabetes increases the risk of cardiovascular and other diseases. When this is taken into account, the attributable mortality for diabetes is at least 1.5 million, and is likely to be considerably higher.

11. Alcohol/drug dependence. Estimates for alcohol and drug dependence represent only a small fraction of the burden of disease and injury attributable to alcohol and drug use. Alcohol and other drug use contributes as a risk factor to a

broad range of diseases, injuries and deaths, other than through dependence.

12. Perinatal conditions. These include low birth weight, birth asphyxia and birth trauma.

ANNEX TABLE 5

All the demographic indicators are based on *World population prospects: The 1998 revision*, New York, United Nations, 1999. Exceptions are: the probability of dying before age 5 for 1978 are based on supplementary tabulations to the 1996 revision of this publication; and the number of deaths and the crude death rate for 1998 are based on Annex Table 2. GDP per capita adjusted for purchasing power, reported in 1985 US$, was taken from the Penn World Table dataset, Mark 5.6, the Chain index (see Note 10, Annex Table 1). All indicators are reported for 1978 and 1998, except for GDP per capita, which is reported for 1978 and 1992 because 1992 is the latest year for which data are available.

ANNEX TABLE 6

Performance measures for each country relate the actual levels of infant mortality and female life expectancy in the indicated year to their predicted level. The predictors used are the logarithm of per capita income (adjusted for purchasing power), the square of the logarithm of per capita income, and indicator variables controlling for time (since, at any income level, health conditions have for the most part substantially improved over this time period). The per capita income figures are from the Penn World Table, Version 5.6 (Heston A, Summers R. International price and quantity comparisons: potentials and pitfalls. *International macro- and microeconomic data,* 1996, **86**: 20–24; see also Note 10, Annex Table 1). The model relating performance to predictors is a random-effects model estimated by generalized least square (STATA (Statistics/Data Analysis). *STATA References.* College Station TX, STATA Corporation, 1996.). Health data are from *World population prospects: The 1998 revision,* New York, United Nations, 1999. More extensive results and a description of the methods are reported in Wang J, Jamison DT, Regression residuals as performance measures: An assessment of robustness in the context of country-level data (paper presented at the annual meeting of the American Educational Research Association, San Diego, 1998), although that document uses World Bank demographic numbers.

The country performance measures on mortality are constructed using regression residuals; Wang & Jamison (1998, above) discuss the use of residuals to measure performance in this context. Based on the derived regression residuals, we constructed performance measures for all countries for which we have data. For infant mortality rates, the performance measures are the percentage by which actual mortality rates exceed predicted rates. For life expectancy, the actual and predicted values are expressed in years. A positive measure of life expectancy means that the observed life expectancy for a certain country is higher than the predicted live expectancy, given one country's income level and the time of the observation. Positive performance measures on infant mortality rate mean worse performance than the prediction.

ANNEX TABLE 7

Estimates of the percentage of the population in each country that lives in absolute poverty are from the World Bank, World Development Indicators 1998 CD-Rom. The definition of absolute poverty used here refers to a per capita income equivalent to less than one international dollar per day. Estimates of the probability of dying in children and adults are for the period 1990–1995 and were taken from *World population prospects: The 1998 revision,* New York, United Nations, 1999. Estimates for tuberculosis prevalence were provided by the Department of Communicable Disease Prevention and Control, Communicable Diseases Cluster, WHO, Geneva.

The analysis was conducted using a methodology for ecological inference developed by Gary King at Harvard University. The methods are described in detail in: Gakidou E, Jamison DT, King G, Spohr C. *Health status of the poor versus the non-poor*, 1999 (forthcoming). The software package – EI – is available for free download at: http://gking.harvard.edu. Background information on the literature on ecological inferences can be found in: King G. *A solution to the ecological inference problem: Reconstructing individual behavior from aggregate data.* Princeton University Press, 1997; and in: King G, Rosen O, Tanner M. Binomial-beta hierarchical models for ecological inference. *Sociological methods and research* (forthcoming), also available at: http://gking.harvard.edu.

Ecological inference, as traditionally defined, is the process of using aggregate data to infer discrete individual-level relationships of interest when individual-level data are not available. In this analysis we have used aggregate data on health measures (probability of adult and child dying, tuberculosis incidence/prevalence) and poverty to infer the magnitude of these health measures in the poor and non-poor subgroups of the populations of these countries. A weighted average estimate is provided as well.

ANNEX TABLE 8

The estimates of malaria for Africa are based on the review by Snow RW, Craig M, Deichmann U, Marsh K (Estimating mortality, morbidity and disability due to malaria among Africa's non-pregnant population. Submitted to the *Bulletin of the World Health Organization,*1999). Estimates for other regions have been prepared by the Global Programme on Evidence for Health Policy and Roll Back Malaria, based on data and information available to WHO.

ANNEX TABLE 9

Source: Global Programme on Evidence for Health Policy, Evidence and Information for Policy Cluster, WHO, Geneva.

ANNEX TABLE 10

Estimates for tuberculosis were provided by the Department of Communicable Disease Prevention and Control, Communicable Diseases Cluster, WHO, Geneva. The methods employed to derive these estimates are described in: Dye C, Scheele S, Dolin P, Pathania V, Raviglione MC. *Global burden of tuberculosis: Estimated incidence, prevalence and mortality by country in 1997* (in press, available from CDC/CPC, WHO, Geneva).

Annex Table 1 Basic indicators for all Member States

Member States by WHO Region[a]	POPULATION						MORTALITY RATES						Maternal mortality ratio (per 100 000)
	Total population		Dependency ratio (per 100)		Total fertility rate		Infant mortality rate (per 1 000)		Probability of dying (per 1 000)				
									under age 5		between age 15 and age 59		
	Size (000)	Annual growth rate (%)							Males	Females	Males	Females	
	1998	1978-1998	1978	1998	1978	1998	1978	1998	1998	1998	1998	1998	1990
All Member States	5 884 576	1.6	72	59	3.9	2.7	87	57	83	83	225	156	430
Africa	601 783	2.8	94	90	6.7	5.4	121	91	172	154	477	428	940
1 Algeria	30 081	2.7	104	70	7.2	3.8	112	44	57	45	147	120	160
2 Angola	12 092	3.0	89	102	6.8	6.8	161	125	217	199	413	355	1 500
3 Benin	5 781	2.9	94	98	7.1	5.8	122	88	142	124	373	318	990
4 Botswana	1 570	3.2	105	83	6.4	4.4	76	59	112	101	676	610	250
5 Burkina Faso	11 305	2.7	100	100	7.8	6.6	127	99	176	166	557	518	930
6 Burundi	6 457	2.5	94	97	6.8	6.3	127	119	189	168	603	545	1 300
7 Cameroon	14 305	2.8	91	90	6.5	5.3	108	74	120	109	389	345	550
8 Cape Verde	408	1.8	110	81	6.7	3.6	86	56	68	60	213	125	...
9 Central African Republic	3 485	2.3	82	88	5.9	4.9	122	98	172	141	580	521	700
10 Chad	7 270	2.7	83	97	6.6	6.1	154	112	184	164	452	400	1 500
11 Comoros	658	3.1	102	85	7.1	4.8	116	76	112	101	303	254	950
12 Congo	2 785	2.9	93	98	6.3	6.1	91	90	147	116	539	475	890
13 Côte d'Ivoire	14 292	3.2	95	88	7.4	5.1	117	87	144	129	555	549	810
14 Democratic Republic of the Congo	49 139	3.4	94*	103	6.5	6.4	117	90	148	130	442	391	870
15 Equatorial Guinea	431	3.7	82	89	5.7	5.6	149	108	184	169	379	322	820
16 Eritrea	3 577	2.3	89	89	6.4	5.7	123	91	154	137	430	374	1 400
17 Ethiopia	59 649	2.8	92	96	6.8	6.3	149	116	193	174	559	528	1 400
18 Gabon	1 167	3.0	67	84	4.4	5.4	122	87	143	127	395	353	500
19 Gambia	1 229	3.6	82	77	6.5	5.2	167	122	212	194	408	350	1 100
20 Ghana	19 162	3.1	92	89	6.5	5.2	99	66	107	95	280	227	740
21 Guinea	7 337	2.7	93	90	7.0	5.5	167	124	207	208	402	366	1 600
22 Guinea-Bissau	1 161	2.3	74	88	5.6	5.8	176	130	214	192	443	391	910
23 Kenya	29 008	3.2	114	90	8.1	4.5	88	66	107	101	515	475	650
24 Lesotho	2 062	2.4	85	79	5.7	4.8	121	93	132	127	362	304	610
25 Liberia	2 666	2.1	92	97	6.8	6.3	167	116	184	163	489	445	560
26 Madagascar	15 057	2.9	94	90	6.6	5.4	130	83	123	110	319	267	490
27 Malawi	10 346	2.9	99	100	7.6	6.8	177	138	223	217	632	599	560
28 Mali	10 694	2.5	96	101	7.1	6.6	180	118	244	227	244	219	1 200
29 Mauritania	2 529	2.7	87	89	6.5	5.5	125	92	155	142	345	290	930
30 Mauritius	1 141	1.0	68	48	3.1	1.9	38	16	22	13	229	111	120
31 Mozambique	18 880	2.5	88	93	6.5	6.3	160	114	193	173	509	461	1 500
32 Namibia	1 660	2.7	87	84	6.0	4.9	98	65	125	119	453	427	370
33 Niger	10 078	3.3	96	103	8.1	6.8	157	115	198	181	393	336	1 200
34 Nigeria	106 409	2.7	95	88	6.9	5.2	109	81	154	140	426	375	1 000
35 Rwanda	6 604	1.6	104	94	8.5	6.2	133	124	213	191	619	578	1 300
36 *Sao Tome and Principe*	*141*	*2.4*	...	...	...	...	...	...	...	...	...	...	...
37 Senegal	9 003	2.7	92	90	7.0	5.6	97	63	117	112	418	317	1 200
38 *Seychelles*	*76*	*1.0*	...	...	...	...	...	...	...	...	...	...	...
39 Sierra Leone	4 568	1.9	85	89	6.5	6.1	192	170	277	248	557	504	1 800
40 South Africa	39 357	2.0	76	64	4.5	3.3	72	59	98	76	507	390	230
41 Swaziland	952	3.0	94	85	6.5	4.7	108	65	109	91	284	220	560
42 Togo	4 397	2.9	91	97	6.6	6.1	117	84	137	120	524	481	640
43 Uganda	20 554	2.6	101	108	6.9	7.1	114	107	181	164	707	675	1 200
44 United Republic of Tanzania	32 102	3.1	100	94	6.8	5.5	113	82	138	123	548	509	770
45 Zambia	8 781	2.5	104	100	7.2	5.6	94	82	149	144	774	724	940
46 Zimbabwe	11 377	2.7	104	82	6.6	3.8	86	69	123	111	713	689	570
The Americas	802 811	1.5	67	57	3.3	2.4	56	28	39	31	197	109	140
47 *Antigua and Barbuda*	*67*	*0.6*	...	...	...	...	...	...	...	...	...	...	...
48 Argentina	36 123	1.4	61	61	3.4	2.6	39	22	28	22	187	95	100

	SOCIAL AND ECONOMIC											HEALTH SERVICES AND FINANCE				
	Life expectancy at birth (years)				GDP per capita adjusted for purchasing power			Average years of education for population aged 25+		Malnutrition stunting among children under age 5 (%)		Children immunized against measles (%)		Health expenditures		
														Total (% of GDP)	Public sector (% of GDP)	Public sector (% of total)
	Males		Females		in 1985 US$	Annual growth rate (%)		Females	Male excess over females	Males around	Females around					
	1978	1998	1978	1998	1992	1962-1992	1982-1992	1990	1990	1995	1995	1987	1997	around 1995	around 1995	around 1995
	60	65	63	69	4 123	2.7	2.5	4.5	2.1	...	...	53	82	5.2	2.6	48
	46	49	49	51	1 261	0.9	-1.9	1.9	1.5	...	...	41	57	3.2	1.7	50
1	57	68	59	70	2 719	2.6	-0.4	1.9	1.9	18	18	59	74	4.6	3.3	73
2	38	45	42	48	...	...	...	...	...	...	...	55	78	...	4.1	...
3	45	52	49	55	...	...	...	0.7	1.2	27	23	26	82	...	1.7	...
4	55	46	58	48	...	...	...	2.4	0.5	...	...	48	79	2.9	1.6	55
5	42	44	44	45	514	0.6	0.0	...	...	35	32	65	68	5.5	2.3	42
6	44	41	48	44	569	0.4	1.2	...	...	...	...	54	...	...	0.8	...
7	47	53	50	56	1 029	1.3	-2.2	1.7	1.3	27	25	...	43	1.4	1.0	72
8	59	66	62	71	1 085	3.0	1.9	...	...	...	...	75	82	...	3.4	...
9	42	43	47	47	514	-1.0	-2.6	...	...	27	30	14	...	...	1.9	...
10	39	46	43	49	408	-2.2	1.0	...	...	41	39	16	30	3.7	3.7	98
11	49	57	53	60	527	-0.2	-2.1	...	...	36	32	71	49	1.2	0.9	79
12	46	46	51	51	2 240	2.3	-1.2	2.9	2.2	...	...	66	18	6.3	3.2	50
13	46	46	50	47	1 104	-0.2	-4.2	...	...	25	24	...	68	3.5	1.4	41
14	46	49	50	52	...	...	...	1.3	2.0	47	44	41	20	...	0.2	...
15	40	48	44	52	...	...	...	...	...	...	...	...	82	6.3	5.2	81
16	44	49	47	52	...	...	...	...	...	36	41	...	53	2.0	1.1	55
17	40	42	44	44	...	...	...	...	...	66	63	13	52	2.6	1.6	61
18	45	51	49	54	3 622	1.8	-1.5	...	...	...	...	67	...	...	0.5	...
19	37	45	41	49	...	...	...	0.5	0.8	33	28	88	91	...	2.0	...
20	50	58	54	62	956	0.1	1.9	1.5	2.6	28	24	28	59	1.5	1.4	94
21	38	46	39	47	740	0.8	-0.6	...	...	...	...	...	56	...	1.2	...
22	36	43	39	46	634	0.8	0.0	...	...	...	...	60	51	...	1.1	...
23	51	51	55	53	914	1.5	0.6	1.9	1.9	35	32	...	32	2.6	1.6	62
24	50	55	54	57	952	3.3	-0.8	3.8	-1.1	46	41	84	53	...	4.1	...
25	48	46	51	49	...	...	...	1.0	1.9	...	...	40	...	...	...	...
26	48	56	51	59	608	-2.2	-3.0	...	...	51	48	27	...	...	1.1	...
27	42	39	44	40	496	0.8	0.0	1.6	1.8	50	47	81	87	...	2.3	...
28	44	52	46	55	...	...	...	0.4	0.8	31	29	8	56	2.7	1.2	46
29	44	52	47	55	837	0.1	-0.6	...	...	...	...	27	20	5.2	1.1	21
30	62	68	68	75	6 167	2.4	4.7	4.4	1.6	...	...	...	...	4.0	2.3	58
31	42	44	45	47	711	-1.8	-2.4	0.4	0.7	...	...	37	70	...	4.6	...
32	50	52	53	53	2 774	1.1	-1.2	...	...	30	27	...	57	7.2	3.7	52
33	39	47	42	50	...	...	...	0.3	0.6	41	38	...	42	...	1.6	...
34	43	49	47	52	978	1.9	-3.7	...	...	43	42	24	69	1.3	0.3	25
35	43	39	47	42	762	1.6	-0.7	0.9	1.2	50	47	74	66	...	1.9	...
36	...	...	...	...	...	...	...	...	...	...	...	69	60	...	6.2	...
37	42	51	46	54	...	...	...	1.3	1.1	24	22	...	65	...	2.5	...
38	...	...	...	...	...	...	...	...	...	...	...	100	100	...	4.0	...
39	34	36	37	39	734	-0.9	-3.7	0.8	1.1	...	...	...	28	3.6	1.5	43
40	52	52	59	58	3 068	1.0	-1.6	4.4	0.8	24	22	75	...	7.9	3.6	45
41	48	58	52	63	...	...	...	3.1	0.9	...	...	77	57	...	2.8	...
42	46	48	50	50	530	1.2	-2.1	1.3	2.5	36	32	57	38	3.4	1.2	35
43	45	39	49	40	547	-0.2	-5.6	0.8	1.2	40	37	48	60	3.9	1.8	45
44	47	47	51	49	...	...	...	...	...	45	42	78	69	...	2.5	...
45	48	40	51	41	...	...	...	2.7	2.8	43	42	65	69	3.3	2.6	78
46	52	44	56	45	1 162	0.7	-1.4	1.7	1.3	...	...	80	73	6.2	2.2	35
	65	69	71	76	9 997	1.9	0.8	7.8	0.6	...	...	66	93	8.6	4.1	47
47	...	...	...	...	...	...	...	...	...	...	...	86	93	5.4	2.9	54
48	65	70	72	77	...	...	...	7.7	0.1	7	2	81	98	9.7	4.3	44

Annex Table 1 Basic indicators for all Member States

Member States by WHO Region[a]	Total population		Dependency ratio (per 100)		Total fertility rate		Infant mortality rate (per 1 000)		Probability of dying (per 1 000) under age 5		between age 15 and age 59		Maternal mortality ratio (per 100 000)
	Size (000)	Annual growth rate (%)							Males	Females	Males	Females	
	1998	1978-1998	1978	1998	1978	1998	1978	1998	1998	1998	1998	1998	1990
All Member States	5 884 576	1.6	72	59	3.9	2.7	87	57	83	83	225	156	430
49 Bahamas	296	1.9	78	56	3.2	2.6	29	16	20	15	207	111	100
50 Barbados	268	0.4	68	50	2.2	1.5	27	12	14	15	126	80	43
51 Belize	230	2.5	106	83	6.2	3.7	45	29	37	37	116	85	...
52 Bolivia	7 957	2.2	86	79	5.8	4.4	131	66	92	83	271	219	650
53 Brazil	165 851	1.8	75	54	4.3	2.3	79	42	54	41	292	157	220
54 Canada	30 563	1.2	49	47	1.8	1.6	12	6	8	6	108	61	6
55 Chile	14 824	1.6	67	56	3.0	2.4	45	13	17	13	158	86	65
56 Colombia	40 803	2.0	84	61	4.3	2.8	57	30	43	35	220	119	100
57 Costa Rica	3 841	2.9	77	62	3.9	2.8	30	12	16	13	124	75	55
58 Cuba	11 116	0.7	71	45	2.1	1.6	23	9	13	10	141	101	95
59 *Dominica*	*71*	*-0.2*	...	...	...	...	...	...	...	...	...	...	...
60 Dominican Republic	8 232	2.1	87	62	4.7	2.8	84	34	51	41	167	121	110
61 Ecuador	12 175	2.4	90	65	5.4	3.1	82	46	66	54	190	127	150
62 El Salvador	6 032	1.6	94	70	5.6	3.2	95	32	45	37	239	153	300
63 *Grenada*	*93*	*0.2*	...	...	...	...	...	...	...	...	...	...	...
64 Guatemala	10 801	2.6	95	91	6.4	4.9	91	46	65	57	312	201	200
65 Guyana	850	0.6	85	54	3.9	2.3	67	58	90	65	262	165	...
66 Haiti	7 952	2.1	85	83	6.0	4.4	139	68	112	97	472	367	1 000
67 Honduras	6 147	3.1	101	85	6.6	4.3	81	35	54	43	208	150	220
68 Jamaica	2 538	1.0	95	64	4.0	2.5	37	22	28	25	132	80	120
69 Mexico	95 831	2.0	99	63	5.3	2.8	57	31	41	34	198	108	110
70 Nicaragua	4 807	2.8	100	88	6.4	4.4	90	43	64	53	217	157	160
71 Panama	2 767	2.0	85	60	4.1	2.6	35	21	29	26	148	96	55
72 Paraguay	5 222	2.9	90	78	5.2	4.2	51	39	54	43	178	120	160
73 Peru	24 797	2.1	86	64	5.4	3.0	99	45	71	58	201	135	280
74 *Saint Kitts and Nevis*	*39*	*-0.7*	...	...	...	...	...	...	...	...	...	...	...
75 *Saint Lucia*	*150*	*1.5*	...	...	...	...	...	...	...	...	...	...	...
76 *Saint Vincent and the Grenadines*	*112*	*0.8*	...	...	...	...	...	...	...	...	...	...	...
77 Suriname	414	0.8	92	60	4.2	2.2	44	29	39	28	210	130	...
78 Trinidad and Tobago	1 283	1.0	69	51	3.4	1.7	32	15	19	12	162	107	90
79 United States of America	274 028	1.0	52	52	1.8	2.0	14	7	10	8	154	79	12
80 Uruguay	3 289	0.7	60	60	2.9	2.4	42	18	23	17	179	92	85
81 Venezuela	23 242	2.5	81	65	4.5	3.0	39	21	27	22	184	105	120
Eastern Mediterranean	473 644	2.8	90	78	6.5	4.4	118	69	107	102	214	172	440
82 Afghanistan	21 354	1.4	85	84	7.2	6.9	183	152	257	257	371	324	1 700
83 Bahrain	595	3.2	67	50	5.2	2.9	43	17	26	17	143	92	60
84 Cyprus	771	1.2	53	55	2.3	2.0	20	9	10	9	115	65	5
85 Djibouti	623	4.7	86	80	6.7	5.3	143	106	182	166	376	319	570
86 Egypt	65 978	2.3	78	68	5.3	3.4	131	51	65	64	201	139	170
87 Iran, Islamic Republic of	65 758	3.0	94	75	6.5	2.8	100	35	52	51	170	150	120
88 Iraq	21 800	3.0	96	82	6.6	5.3	84	95	119	114	243	192	310
89 Jordan	6 304	4.3	108	82	7.4	4.9	65	26	32	31	185	142	150
90 Kuwait	1 811	2.0	77	61	5.9	2.9	34	12	16	14	103	68	29
91 Lebanon	3 191	0.8	85	64	4.3	2.7	48	29	39	31	180	133	300
92 Libyan Arab Jamahiriya	5 339	3.3	95	73	7.4	3.8	63	28	32	31	189	143	220
93 Morocco	27 377	2.0	95	61	5.9	3.1	110	51	74	62	193	142	610
94 Oman	2 382	4.3	89	90	7.2	5.9	95	25	35	24	170	115	190
95 Pakistan	148 166	3.1	92	83	7.0	5.0	130	74	108	104	192	148	340
96 Qatar	579	5.4	53	39	6.1	3.7	46	17	27	18	150	82	...
97 Saudi Arabia	20 181	4.4	90	78	7.3	5.8	75	23	31	24	157	114	130
98 Somalia	9 237	2.9	98	101	7.3	7.3	149	122	212	195	408	350	1 600

	SOCIAL AND ECONOMIC											HEALTH SERVICES AND FINANCE				
	Life expectancy at birth (years)				GDP per capita adjusted for purchasing power			Average years of education for population aged 25+		Malnutrition stunting among children under age 5 (%)		Children immunized against measles (%)		Health expenditures		
	Males		Females		in 1985 US$	Annual growth rate (%)		Females	Male excess over females	Males around	Females around			Total (% of GDP) around	Public sector (% of GDP) around	Public sector (% of total) around
	1978	1998	1978	1998	1992	1962-1992	1982-1992	1990	1990	1995	1995	1987	1997	1995	1995	1995
	60	65	63	69	4 123	2.7	2.5	4.5	2.1	...	...	53	82	5.2	2.6	48
49	63	71	71	77	...	...	...	...	...	...	...	...	93	4.2	2.5	59
50	69	74	74	79	...	...	...	8.2	0.0	...	...	...	92	6.8	4.4	65
51	69	73	71	76	4 253	...	1.8	...	...	...	...	64	98	8.0	6.0	75
52	48	60	52	63	1 721	1.2	-0.8	3.3	1.7	33	26	33	98	7.1	4.1	58
53	60	63	64	71	3 882	2.4	-0.2	3.5	0.1	12	9	63	99	4.6	1.8	40
54	71	76	78	82	16 362	2.6	1.8	10.2	0.3	...	...	70	...	9.2	6.6	71
55	64	72	71	78	4 890	1.6	3.5	6.1	0.1	...	...	92	92	6.2	2.5	40
56	62	67	66	74	3 380	2.2	1.4	4.5	-0.6	16	14	72	89	7.4	2.9	40
57	69	74	73	79	3 569	1.7	1.5	5.3	0.1	6	7	90	99	8.5	6.3	74
58	71	74	75	78	...	...	...	6.4	0.5	...	...	99	99	...	7.9	...
59	...	...	...	...	...	...	...	...	...	...	...	87	99	6.3	4.0	63
60	60	69	64	73	2 250	1.7	0.0	3.5	0.5	12	9	71	80	5.7	1.8	32
61	60	67	63	72	2 830	2.2	-1.2	5.3	0.7	...	...	46	75	5.3	2.0	39
62	52	67	62	73	1 876	0.6	0.7	3.0	0.8	23	24	48	97	5.9	2.4	41
63	...	...	...	...	...	...	...	...	...	...	...	77	92	5.2	2.8	53
64	54	61	58	67	2 247	0.9	-0.4	2.2	0.7	50	49	24	74	3.2	1.7	54
65	58	61	63	68	...	...	...	5.4	-0.1	...	...	52	82	5.2	4.3	83
66	49	51	52	56	...	...	...	1.3	1.8	32	32	24	...	3.6	1.3	40
67	56	68	60	72	1 385	0.9	-0.4	3.6	0.2	39	40	69	89	5.6	2.8	50
68	68	73	72	77	...	...	...	4.8	-0.6	...	...	62	88	4.9	2.5	51
69	62	70	69	75	6 253	2.6	0.5	5.4	0.9	23	23	54	97	4.2	2.4	56
70	55	66	60	71	...	...	...	3.1	0.5	25	22	44	94	8.6	5.3	61
71	67	72	71	76	3 332	2.1	-0.8	7.6	-0.2	...	...	78	92	6.7	4.7	70
72	64	67	69	72	2 178	1.9	-1.0	4.5	0.5	14	14	56	61	5.1	1.8	36
73	57	66	60	71	2 092	-0.3	-3.5	5.0	0.9	26	25	35	94	3.7	2.2	60
74	...	...	...	...	4 799	...	...	...	...	...	...	91	97	5.3	3.2	61
75	...	...	...	...	...	...	...	...	...	...	...	81	95	3.8	2.5	66
76	...	...	...	...	...	...	...	...	...	...	...	91	99	7.0	5.2	74
77	63	68	68	73	...	...	...	...	...	...	...	70	78	4.0	2.0	50
78	66	72	71	76	...	...	...	6.2	0.1	...	...	68	88	3.4	2.1	61
79	69	73	77	80	17 945	1.8	1.9	11.6	0.9	2	2	82	...	14.0	6.6	47
80	66	70	73	78	5 185	1.0	1.1	6.9	-0.4	10	9	99	80	13.4	7.0	52
81	65	70	71	76	7 082	0.2	0.3	4.8	0.2	15	12	57	68	7.5	3.0	40
	53	63	55	65	2 139	2.2	1.3	1.7	2.2	...	...	57	83	3.6	1.6	38
82	40	45	40	46	...	...	...	0.3	1.4	54	49	31	58	...	...	...
83	64	71	68	75	...	...	...	4.3	0.5	...	...	73	95	7.0	...	...
84	72	76	76	80	9 203	4.5	5.1	7.2	1.2	...	...	91	90	4.6	...	...
85	41	49	45	52	...	...	...	...	...	...	...	22	59	...	...	...
86	53	65	55	68	1 869	2.6	0.8	2.3	2.7	26	23	76	92	3.7	1.6	43
87	58	69	59	70	3 685	0.8	-0.5	2.3	1.9	20	18	62	96	4.8	2.8	58
88	61	61	62	64	...	...	...	2.0	2.3	...	...	66	98	...	...	...
89	59	69	63	72	...	...	...	3.8	2.7	16	16	80	95	7.9	3.7	47
90	68	74	72	78	...	...	...	5.7	0.0	...	...	95	95	...	3.6	...
91	63	68	67	72	...	...	...	...	...	13	12	81	89	5.3	2.1	39
92	56	68	59	72	...	...	...	...	...	16	14	56	92	...	...	...
93	54	65	58	69	2 173	2.3	1.1	...	...	24	24	73	92	3.4	1.6	48
94	54	69	56	73	...	...	...	...	...	19	13	86	98	...	2.5	...
95	53	63	54	65	1 432	2.6	2.4	1.0	2.5	...	...	52	74	3.5	0.8	22
96	64	70	68	75	...	...	...	...	...	8	8	62	87	2.8	...	...
97	58	70	60	73	...	...	...	...	...	...	...	77	92	3.1	...	...
98	40	45	44	49	...	...	...	...	...	...	...	29	...	...	...	...

Annex Table 1 Basic indicators for all Member States

Member States by WHO Region[a]	POPULATION							MORTALITY RATES						Maternal mortality ratio (per 100 000)
	Total population		Dependency ratio (per 100)		Total fertility rate			Infant mortality rate (per 1 000)		Probability of dying (per 1 000)				
										under age 5		between age 15 and age 59		
	Size (000)	Annual growth rate (%)								Males	Females	Males	Females	
	1998	1978-1998	1978	1998	1978	1998	1978	1998		1998	1998	1998	1998	1990
All Member States	5 884 576	1.6	72	59	3.9	2.7	87	57		83	83	225	156	430
99 Sudan	28 292	2.4	91	77	6.7	4.6	97	71		115	108	357	302	660
100 Syrian Arab Republic	15 333	3.2	108	84	7.4	4.0	67	33		47	33	197	138	180
101 Tunisia	9 335	2.1	86	60	5.7	2.6	88	30		38	36	176	144	170
102 United Arab Emirates	2 353	5.6	43	46	5.7	3.4	38	16		21	17	99	65	26
103 Yemen	16 887	4.0	115	102	7.6	7.6	158	80		112	114	303	274	1 400
Europe	870 128	0.5	56	50	2.2	1.6	35	21		30	23	217	95	59
104 Albania	3 119	1.0	73	57	4.2	2.5	50	30		46	39	122	65	65
105 *Andorra*	72	4.4	...	...	...	...	...	...		...	...	...	...	...
106 Armenia	3 536	0.8	60	53	2.5	1.7	22	26		35	30	222	115	50
107 Austria	8 140	0.4	59	47	1.6	1.4	17	6		8	7	137	63	10
108 Azerbaijan	7 669	1.3	73	58	3.6	2.0	41	36		55	44	243	111	22
109 Belarus	10 315	0.4	52	50	2.1	1.4	22	23		36	20	339	126	37
110 Belgium	10 141	0.2	54	51	1.7	1.6	14	7		9	7	119	64	10
111 Bosnia and Herzegovina	3 675	-0.2	53	41	2.2	1.4	36	15		19	15	172	88	...
112 Bulgaria	8 336	-0.3	51	48	2.2	1.2	22	17		23	16	225	99	27
113 Croatia	4 481	0.2	49	47	2.0	1.6	21	10		14	11	213	86	...
114 Czech Republic	10 282	0.0	57	45	2.3	1.2	18	6		9	7	183	81	15
115 Denmark	5 270	0.2	56	49	1.7	1.7	9	7		10	7	141	96	9
116 Estonia	1 429	-0.1	52	47	2.1	1.3	22	19		33	17	314	109	41
117 Finland	5 154	0.4	48	49	1.6	1.7	9	6		7	6	151	58	11
118 France	58 683	0.5	58	53	1.9	1.7	11	6		8	7	145	63	15
119 Georgia	5 059	0.1	55	54	2.4	1.9	36	20		27	20	221	86	33
120 Germany	82 133	0.2	54	47	1.5	1.3	15	5		7	6	132	66	22
121 Greece	10 600	0.6	57	49	2.3	1.3	25	8		9	8	110	49	10
122 Hungary	10 116	-0.3	53	47	2.1	1.4	27	10		13	10	281	128	30
123 Iceland	276	1.0	62	53	2.3	2.1	9	5		6	6	92	63	0
124 Ireland	3 681	0.5	72	50	3.5	1.9	15	7		9	7	114	66	10
125 Israel	5 984	2.4	71	61	3.4	2.7	18	8		11	9	102	61	7
126 Italy	57 369	0.1	56	47	1.9	1.2	18	7		9	8	108	54	12
127 Kazakhstan	16 319	0.6	64	55	3.1	2.3	45	35		46	36	306	133	80
128 Kyrgyzstan	4 643	1.4	78	72	4.1	3.2	55	40		56	44	282	135	110
129 Latvia	2 424	-0.2	51	49	2.0	1.3	23	18		31	18	334	118	40
130 Lithuania	3 694	0.4	55	50	2.1	1.4	22	21		29	18	309	111	36
131 Luxembourg	422	0.7	50	48	1.5	1.7	13	7		8	8	130	62	0
132 Malta	384	1.0	50	48	2.0	1.9	15	8		11	8	93	55	...
133 *Monaco*	33	1.2	...	...	...	...	...	...		...	...	...	...	...
134 Netherlands	15 678	0.6	53	47	1.6	1.5	10	6		9	7	102	65	12
135 Norway	4 419	0.4	59	54	1.8	1.9	9	5		7	6	107	59	6
136 Poland	38 718	0.5	51	48	2.3	1.5	23	15		18	14	224	88	19
137 Portugal	9 869	0.2	59	47	2.4	1.4	30	9		12	10	156	72	15
138 Republic of Moldova	4 378	0.5	53	52	2.4	1.8	46	29		39	25	302	156	60
139 Romania	22 474	0.1	57	46	2.6	1.2	31	23		39	26	243	105	130
140 Russian Federation	147 434	0.4	47	46	1.9	1.3	30	18		25	19	400	146	75
141 *San Marino*	26	1.2	...	...	...	...	...	...		...	...	...	...	...
142 Slovakia	5 377	0.5	57	47	2.5	1.4	22	11		14	12	216	89	...
143 Slovenia	1 993	0.5	54	43	2.2	1.3	17	7		9	8	189	81	13
144 Spain	39 628	0.4	60	46	2.6	1.2	16	7		9	7	129	54	7
145 Sweden	8 875	0.4	56	56	1.6	1.6	8	5		7	6	97	63	7
146 Switzerland	7 299	0.7	52	47	1.5	1.5	10	6		10	7	114	60	6
147 Tajikistan	6 015	2.4	94	84	5.9	4.2	69	57		88	73	219	142	130

#	|	Life expectancy at birth (years)				GDP per capita adjusted for purchasing power			Average years of education for population aged 25+		Malnutrition stunting among children under age 5 (%)		|	Children immunized against measles (%)		Health expenditures		
		Males		Females		in 1985 US$	Annual growth rate (%)		Females	Male excess over females	Males around 1995	Females around 1995				Total (% of GDP) around 1995	Public sector (% of GDP) around 1995	Public sector (% of total) around 1995
		1978	1998	1978	1998	1992	1962-1992	1982-1992	1990	1990				1987	1997			
		60	65	63	69	4 123	2.7	2.5	4.5	2.1	...	...		53	82	5.2	2.6	48
99		45	54	48	56	...	...	...	0.6	1.2	34	34		22	92	0.3	...	...
100		58	67	62	71	...	...	...	2.9	3.0	23	18		63	93	...	...	...
101		60	68	61	71	3 075	3.5	1.7	2.0	2.0	22	23		74	92	5.9	3.0	52
102		65	74	69	76	...	...	...	...	...	...	...		56	95	2.5	2.0	81
103		44	57	44	58	...	...	...	...	...	36	47		22	51	2.5	1.1	43
		67	69	74	77	10 189	2.6	2.0	6.9	0.8	...	...		65	87	7.1	5.2	78
104		67	70	71	76	...	...	...	...	...	...	...		96	95	...	2.5	...
105		...	...	...	...	...	...	...	...	...	...	...		...	90	...	...	...
106		69	67	75	74	...	...	...	...	...	...	...		...	92	7.8	3.1	40
107		69	74	76	80	12 955	2.9	2.1	6.6	1.9	...	...		60	90	8.0	6.0	75
108		64	66	72	74	...	...	...	...	...	24	20		...	...	6.1	1.1	19
109		66	62	76	74	...	...	...	...	...	...	...		...	98	6.4	5.3	83
110		69	74	76	81	13 484	2.7	2.1	8.4	0.7	...	...		50	64	7.9	6.9	88
111		67	71	72	76	...	...	...	...	...	...	...		...	85	...	...	...
112		69	68	74	75	5 208	...	2.0	9.0	0.5	...	...		100	93	6.9	5.5	80
113		67	69	74	77	...	...	...	...	...	...	...		...	93	10.1	8.5	84
114		67	70	74	77	...	...	...	...	...	2	2		...	96	9.1	7.4	81
115		71	73	77	78	14 091	2.1	2.0	10.9	0.7	...	...		82	84	6.4	5.1	79
116		65	63	74	75	...	...	...	...	...	...	...		...	88	...	6.4	...
117		68	73	77	81	12 000	2.5	0.7	9.6	0.3	...	...		...	...	7.5	5.6	75
118		70	74	78	82	13 918	2.6	1.5	6.6	0.7	...	...		41	83	9.7	7.8	81
119		67	69	74	77	...	...	...	...	...	...	...		...	95	...	0.6	...
120		69	74	76	80	...	...	...	...	...	...	...		50	...	10.5	8.2	78
121		72	76	76	81	...	...	...	6.4	2.7	...	...		81	90	5.9	4.9	83
122		66	67	73	75	4 645	...	-1.1	8.0	0.9	...	...		100	100	7.3	6.8	93
123		73	77	79	81	12 618	3.0	0.5	7.6	0.7	...	...		...	...	8.0	6.7	84
124		70	74	75	79	9 637	3.3	3.2	8.1	0.0	...	...		...	...	6.4	5.1	81
125		71	76	75	80	9 843	3.1	1.9	8.7	0.7	...	...		89	94	4.1	...	...
126		70	75	77	81	12 721	3.0	2.2	5.7	1.0	...	...		21	75	7.6	5.3	70
127		60	63	70	72	...	...	...	...	...	18	14		...	97	...	2.2	...
128		60	63	68	72	...	...	...	...	...	...	...		...	98	...	3.5	...
129		64	62	74	74	...	...	...	...	...	...	...		...	97	...	4.4	...
130		66	64	75	76	...	...	...	...	...	...	...		...	96	...	4.8	...
131		68	73	75	80	16 798	2.3	3.5	...	...	...	...		77	91	7.0	6.5	93
132		70	75	74	79	...	...	...	6.3	0.8	...	...		59	...	7.4	...	...
133		...	...	...	...	...	...	...	...	...	...	...		...	...	...	...	...
134		72	75	79	81	13 281	2.5	2.0	8.2	0.8	...	...		93	96	8.6	6.6	77
135		72	75	79	81	15 518	3.2	2.5	7.6	0.8	...	...		87	...	7.9	6.5	83
136		67	68	75	77	3 826	...	0.5	9.3	0.6	...	...		94	...	6.0	5.0	83
137		67	72	74	79	...	...	...	3.3	0.7	...	...		81	...	8.2	4.9	60
138		62	64	69	72	...	...	...	...	...	...	...		...	99	...	4.9	...
139		67	66	72	74	...	...	...	8.6	1.3	8	8		90	97	...	3.6	...
140		62	61	73	73	...	...	...	...	...	12	13		92	...	4.8	4.1	87
141		...	...	...	...	...	...	...	...	...	...	...		...	...	...	...	...
142		67	69	74	77	...	...	...	...	...	...	...		...	98	...	4.6	...
143		67	71	75	78	...	...	...	...	...	...	...		...	82	...	7.3	...
144		71	75	77	82	9 802	3.2	3.0	6.1	0.4	...	...		85	...	7.7	5.9	76
145		72	76	78	81	13 986	1.8	1.1	9.3	0.4	...	...		93	...	7.3	5.9	80
146		72	75	79	82	15 887	1.4	1.2	8.3	1.2	...	...		...	...	9.8	7.0	72
147		62	64	67	70	...	...	...	...	...	...	...		...	95	...	5.8	...

Annex Table 1 Basic indicators for all Member States

Member States by WHO Region[a]	POPULATION						MORTALITY RATES						Maternal mortality ratio (per 100 000)
	Total population		Dependency ratio (per 100)		Total fertility rate		Infant mortality rate (per 1 000)		Probability of dying (per 1 000)				
									under age 5		between age 15 and age 59		
	Size (000)	Annual growth rate (%)							Males	Females	Males	Females	
	1998	1978-1998	1978	1998	1978	1998	1978	1998	1998	1998	1998	1998	1990
All Member States	5 884 576	1.6	72	59	3.9	2.7	87	57	83	83	225	156	430
148 The Former Yugoslav Republic of Macedonia	1 999	0.7	57	50	2.7	2.1	57	23	37	33	272	173	...
149 Turkey	64 479	2.1	80	53	4.5	2.5	120	45	67	52	174	111	180
150 Turkmenistan	4 309	2.3	87	75	5.3	3.6	73	55	86	69	267	154	55
151 Ukraine	50 861	0.1	50	49	2.0	1.4	23	19	30	20	311	124	50
152 United Kingdom	58 649	0.2	58	54	1.7	1.7	14	7	9	8	110	69	9
153 Uzbekistan	23 574	2.2	89	76	5.1	3.4	58	44	69	56	245	145	55
154 Yugoslavia	10 635	0.6	52	50	2.4	1.8	38	18	28	23	157	77	...
South-East Asia	1 485 056	1.9	79	62	4.9	2.9	121	68	87	97	237	189	610
155 Bangladesh	124 774	2.0	98	67	6.7	3.1	137	79	106	116	295	276	850
156 Bhutan	2 004	2.3	81	88	5.9	5.5	130	63	98	94	268	225	1 600
157 Democratic People's Republic of Korea	23 348	1.5	82	48	3.3	2.1	38	22	27	25	184	108	70
158 India	982 223	2.0	76	64	4.8	3.1	129	72	82	97	230	182	570
159 Indonesia	206 338	1.8	81	56	4.7	2.6	105	48	69	56	236	184	650
160 Maldives	271	3.0	86	91	7.0	5.4	106	50	53	80	208	222	...
161 Myanmar	44 497	1.6	78	51	5.3	2.4	114	79	121	104	262	207	580
162 Nepal	22 847	2.6	85	83	6.2	4.5	142	83	110	124	301	287	1 500
163 Sri Lanka	18 455	1.3	69	51	3.8	2.1	41	18	22	20	171	93	140
164 Thailand	60 300	1.5	83	47	4.3	1.7	56	29	27	24	146	81	200
Western Pacific	1 651 154	1.3	71	49	3.3	1.9	53	38	43	50	162	100	120
165 Australia	18 520	1.3	55	50	2.1	1.8	13	6	8	6	105	56	9
166 Brunei Darussalam	315	2.8	74	58	4.4	2.8	23	10	11	11	124	64	60
167 Cambodia	10 716	2.4	76	82	4.1	4.6	263	103	141	127	400	323	900
168 China	1 255 698	1.3	73	47	3.3	1.8	52	41	43	54	164	101	95
169 *Cook Islands*	*19*	*0.2*	...	...	...	...	...	...	...	...	...	...	...
170 Fiji	796	1.3	72	59	4.0	2.7	37	20	28	18	148	97	90
171 Japan	126 281	0.5	48	45	1.8	1.4	9	4	6	5	99	50	18
172 *Kiribati*	*81*	*1.6*	...	...	...	...	...	...	...	...	...	...	...
173 Lao People's Democratic Republic	5 163	2.5	81	91	6.7	5.8	135	93	154	146	344	296	650
174 Malaysia	21 410	2.5	78	64	4.2	3.2	34	11	16	13	179	107	80
175 *Marshall Islands*	*60*	*3.1*	...	...	...	...	...	...	...	...	...	...	...
176 *Micronesia, Federated States of*	*114*	*1.9*	...	...	...	...	...	...	...	...	...	...	...
177 Mongolia	2 579	2.5	86	67	6.6	2.6	88	51	72	75	224	166	65
178 *Nauru*	*11*	*2.3*	...	...	...	...	...	...	...	...	...	...	...
179 New Zealand	3 796	1.0	60	53	2.2	2.0	14	7	9	8	125	79	26
180 *Niue*	*2*	*-3.2*	...	...	...	...	...	...	...	...	...	...	...
181 *Palau*	*19*	*2.4*	...	...	...	...	...	...	...	...	...	...	...
182 Papua New Guinea	4 600	2.3	81	72	5.9	4.6	77	61	79	88	370	327	930
183 Philippines	72 944	2.3	82	69	5.0	3.6	62	36	49	38	200	151	280
184 Republic of Korea	46 109	1.1	64	40	2.9	1.7	30	10	13	13	203	98	130
185 Samoa	174	0.6	99	76	6.2	4.2	76	23	25	29	178	125	35
186 Singapore	3 476	2.0	51	41	1.9	1.7	13	5	6	6	118	78	10
187 Solomon Islands	417	3.5	106	86	7.1	4.9	47	23	32	22	160	108	...
188 *Tonga*	*98*	*0.4*	...	...	...	...	...	...	...	...	...	...	...
189 *Tuvalu*	*11*	*2.2*	...	...	...	...	...	...	...	...	...	...	...
190 Vanuatu	182	2.5	91	83	5.5	4.3	84	39	54	42	211	157	280
191 Viet Nam	77 562	2.1	91	66	5.6	2.6	82	38	54	57	218	147	160

[a] Italics indicate less populous Member States (under 150 000 population in 1998).

... Data not available or not applicable.

	Life expectancy at birth (years)				GDP per capita adjusted for purchasing power			Average years of education for population aged 25+		Malnutrition stunting among children under age 5 (%)		Children immunized against measles (%)		Health expenditures		
	Males		Females		in 1985 US$	Annual growth rate (%)		Females	Male excess over females	Males around	Females around			Total (% of GDP) around	Public sector (% of GDP) around	Public sector (% of total) around
	1978	1998	1978	1998	1992	1962-1992	1982-1992	1990	1990	1995	1995	1987	1997	1995	1995	1995
	60	65	63	69	4 123	2.7	2.5	4.5	2.1	...	...	53	82	5.2	2.6	48
148	68	71	71	75	...	...	...	...	...	...	...	...	98	8.3	7.3	89
149	58	67	63	72	3 807	2.8	2.9	2.6	1.6	21	20	50	76	4.2	2.7	65
150	58	62	65	69	...	...	...	...	...	...	...	...	100	...	1.2	...
151	64	64	74	74	...	...	...	...	...	...	...	...	...	...	4.9	...
152	70	75	76	80	12 724	2.0	2.2	8.7	0.1	...	...	76	95	6.9	5.8	84
153	62	64	68	71	...	...	...	...	...	34	29	...	88	...	3.5	...
154	68	70	73	75	...	...	...	6.2	2.1	7	7	92	91	...	...	...
	53	62	53	64	1 558	2.2	3.3	2.4	2.3	...	...	40	85	4.7	1.1	27
155	47	58	46	58	1 510	1.5	2.5	1.2	2.1	54	55	6	97	2.4	1.2	48
156	45	60	47	62	...	...	...	...	...	...	...	52	84	...	2.3	...
157	62	69	69	75	...	...	...	...	...	...	...	94	...	...	...	...
158	53	62	52	63	1 282	1.8	3.2	2.2	2.7	52	52	44	81	5.6	1.2	22
159	52	63	54	67	2 102	4.0	3.5	3.2	1.5	43	41	46	92	1.8	0.6	37
160	56	66	53	63	...	...	...	...	...	28	26	41	96	...	4.9	...
161	50	59	53	62	...	...	...	1.8	0.7	47	42	17	88	...	0.4	...
162	47	58	45	57	...	...	...	0.3	1.5	47	50	37	85	5.0	1.2	24
163	65	71	69	75	2 215	1.9	2.1	5.0	0.9	23	25	55	94	1.9	1.4	76
164	59	66	63	72	3 942	4.7	6.0	4.8	0.8	...	...	52	...	5.3	1.4	26
	64	68	67	73	2 959	4.0	4.1	4.4	3.0	...	...	62	94	4.2	2.3	54
165	70	75	77	81	14 458	2.0	1.8	9.8	0.7	...	...	68	87	8.6	5.7	67
166	68	73	71	78	...	...	...	...	...	...	...	100	98	...	2.2	...
167	30	51	33	55	...	...	...	...	...	...	...	52	68	7.2	0.7	10
168	64	68	66	72	1 493	4.1	4.5	3.4	3.6	32	31	63	96	3.8	2.1	54
169	...	...	...	...	...	...	...	...	...	...	...	84	89	...	...	...
170	66	71	69	75	...	...	...	7.0	0.9	2	4	64	75	3.4	2.3	68
171	73	77	78	83	15 105	4.9	3.6	8.8	0.8	...	...	...	...	7.2	5.6	78
172	...	...	...	...	...	...	...	...	...	...	...	14	82	...	22.8	...
173	42	52	45	55	...	...	...	...	...	48	47	11	67	2.6	1.3	48
174	64	70	67	74	5 746	4.5	3.3	4.4	2.3	...	...	41	84	2.5	1.5	60
175	...	...	...	...	...	...	...	...	...	...	...	31	52	...	12.4	...
176	...	...	...	...	...	...	...	...	...	...	...	69	74	...	...	...
177	55	64	58	67	...	...	...	...	...	26	27	61	98	4.7	4.4	92
178	...	...	...	...	...	...	...	...	...	...	...	...	121	...	...	...
179	69	74	76	80	11 363	1.1	0.4	10.8	0.9	...	...	67	114	7.2	5.5	76
180	...	...	...	...	...	...	...	...	...	...	...	94	100	...	...	...
181	...	...	...	...	...	...	...	...	...	...	...	98	83	...	...	...
182	50	57	50	59	1 606	0.4	-0.3	1.2	1.0	...	...	37	40	...	2.8	...
183	58	67	61	70	1 689	1.1	-1.2	6.8	-0.2	34	31	68	90	2.4	1.3	56
184	61	69	68	76	...	...	...	8.1	2.4	...	...	82	85	5.4	...	34
185	61	69	64	74	...	...	...	...	...	...	...	78	99	...	3.1	...
186	69	75	73	79	12 653	6.7	4.8	5.0	1.0	...	...	94	90	3.5	1.3	37
187	63	70	67	74	...	...	...	...	...	...	...	58	68	5.6	4.8	86
188	...	...	...	...	...	...	...	...	...	...	...	88	97	...	4.0	...
189	...	...	...	...	...	...	...	...	...	...	...	65	100	...	...	...
190	55	66	59	70	...	...	...	...	...	...	...	34	65	...	3.3	...
191	54	65	58	70	...	...	...	...	...	47	47	42	96	5.2	1.1	22

Annex Table 2 Mortality by sex, cause and WHO Region, estimates for 1998

DISEASE	WHO MEMBER STATES									
	Both sexes		Males		Females		High income		Low and middle income	
Population (000)	5 884 576		2 963 656		2 920 920		907 828		4 976 748	
	(000)	% total	(000)	% total	(000)	% total	(000)	% total	(000)	% total
TOTAL DEATHS	53 929	100	28 510	100	25 420	100	8 033	100	45 897	100
I. Communicable diseases, maternal and perinatal conditions and nutritional deficiencies	16 447	30.5	8 286	29.1	8 161	32.1	510	6.3	15 937	34.7
A. Infectious and parasitic diseases	9 802	18.2	5 153	18.1	4 649	18.3	122	1.5	9 680	21.1
1. Tuberculosis	1 498	2.8	893	3.1	605	2.4	18	0.2	1 480	3.2
2. STDs excluding HIV	181	0.3	80	0.3	101	0.4	1	0.0	180	0.4
a. Syphilis	159	0.3	80	0.3	80	0.3	1	0.0	159	0.3
b. Chlamydia	13	0.0	0	0.0	13	0.1	0	0.0	13	0.0
c. Gonorrhoea	8	0.0	0	0.0	8	0.0	0	0.0	8	0.0
d. Other STDs	1	0.0	0	0.0	0	0.0	0	0.0	0	0.0
3. HIV/AIDS	2 285	4.2	1 164	4.1	1 121	4.4	32	0.4	2 253	4.9
4. Diarrhoeal diseases	2 219	4.1	1 149	4.0	1 070	4.2	7	0.1	2 212	4.8
5. Childhood diseases	1 650	3.1	846	3.0	804	3.2	10	0.1	1 640	3.6
a. Pertussis	346	0.6	178	0.6	168	0.7	3	0.0	342	0.7
b. Poliomyelitis	2	0.0	1	0.0	1	0.0	0	0.0	2	0.0
c. Diphtheria	5	0.0	3	0.0	2	0.0	0	0.0	5	0.0
d. Measles	888	1.6	456	1.6	432	1.7	5	0.1	882	1.9
e. Tetanus	410	0.8	208	0.7	202	0.8	1	0.0	409	0.9
6. Meningitis	143	0.3	74	0.3	69	0.3	4	0.1	139	0.3
7. Hepatitis	92	0.2	55	0.2	37	0.1	4	0.1	88	0.2
8. Malaria	1 110	2.1	572	2.0	538	2.1	0	0.0	1 110	2.4
9. Tropical diseases	106	0.2	58	0.2	48	0.2	0	0.0	106	0.2
a. Trypanosomiasis	40	0.1	20	0.1	21	0.1	0	0.0	40	0.1
b. Chagas disease	17	0.0	8	0.0	9	0.0	0	0.0	17	0.0
c. Schistosomiasis	7	0.0	4	0.0	3	0.0	0	0.0	7	0.0
d. Leishmaniasis	42	0.1	26	0.1	16	0.1	0	0.0	42	0.1
e. Lymphatic filariasis	0	0.0	0	0.0	0	0.0	0	0.0	0	0.0
f. Onchocerciasis	0	0.0	0	0.0	0	0.0	0	0.0	0	0.0
10. Leprosy	2	0.0	1	0.0	1	0.0	0	0.0	2	0.0
11. Dengue	15	0.0	7	0.0	8	0.0	0	0.0	15	0.0
12. Japanese encephalitis	3	0.0	2	0.0	2	0.0	0	0.0	3	0.0
13. Trachoma	0	0.0	0	0.0	0	0.0	0	0.0	0	0.0
14. Intestinal nematode infections	17	0.0	9	0.0	8	0.0	0	0.0	17	0.0
a. Ascariasis	8	0.0	4	0.0	4	0.0	0	0.0	8	0.0
b. Trichuriasis	5	0.0	3	0.0	2	0.0	0	0.0	5	0.0
c. Hookworm disease	4	0.0	2	0.0	2	0.0	0	0.0	4	0.0
d. Other intestinal infections	0	0.0	0	0.0	0	0.0	0	0.0	0	0.0
15. Other infectious diseases	478	0.9	243	0.9	235	0.9	46	0.6	432	0.9
B. Respiratory infections	3 507	6.5	1 781	6.2	1 726	6.8	309	3.9	3 198	7.0
1. Acute lower respiratory infections	3 452	6.4	1 753	6.1	1 699	6.7	306	3.8	3 146	6.9
2. Acute upper respiratory infections	34	0.1	17	0.1	17	0.1	3	0.0	31	0.1
3. Otitis media	20	0.0	10	0.0	10	0.0	0	0.0	20	0.0
C. Maternal conditions	493	0.9	0	0.0	493	1.9	2	0.0	491	1.1
1. Haemorrhage	123	0.2	0	0.0	123	0.5	0	0.0	122	0.3
2. Sepsis	74	0.1	0	0.0	74	0.3	0	0.0	74	0.2
3. Hypertensive disorders of pregnancy	62	0.1	0	0.0	62	0.2	1	0.0	61	0.1

	AFR	AMR		EMR	EUR		SEAR		WPR		
		High income	**Low and middle income**		**High income**	**Low and middle income**	**India**	**Other low and middle income**	**High income**	**China**	**Other low and middle income**
	601 783	*304 886*	*497 925*	*473 644*	*392 402*	*477 727*	*982 223*	*502 833*	*198 497*	*1 255 698*	*196 958*
	(000)	(000)	(000)	(000)	(000)	(000)	(000)	(000)	(000)	(000)	(000)
	9 621	2 538	3 113	3 773	3 974	5 281	9 337	4 147	1 482	9 296	1 367
I.	6 344	154	726	1 487	239	496	3 944	1 415	108	1 055	479
A.	4 695	38	366	752	51	183	2 121	839	29	456	273
1.	209	1	53	139	7	53	421	261	10	259	86
2.	69	0	9	12	0	2	55	23	0	1	9
a.	62	0	8	11	0	2	47	20	0	0	8
b.	4	0	1	0	0	0	5	2	0	0	1
c.	3	0	0	0	0	0	3	1	0	0	0
d.	0	0	0	0	0	0	0	0	0	0	0
3.	1 830	19	80	16	12	4	179	119	2	8	16
4.	731	1	111	278	4	58	711	183	0	66	76
5.	738	0	31	199	2	32	429	139	7	29	44
a.	130	0	16	50	1	14	71	36	3	13	12
b.	1	0	0	0	0	0	1	0	0	0	0
c.	1	0	0	0	0	1	2	1	0	0	0
d.	503	0	0	96	1	6	190	66	4	5	17
e.	103	0	14	52	1	11	165	37	0	12	15
6.	21	1	12	12	2	8	36	14	1	32	5
7.	13	1	4	8	2	4	16	12	1	28	4
8.	961	0	4	53	0	0	20	53	0	0	20
9.	49	0	18	6	0	1	30	2	0	1	1
a.	38	0	0	3	0	0	0	0	0	0	0
b.	0	0	17	0	0	0	0	0	0	0	0
c.	3	0	0	1	0	0	0	0	0	1	0
d.	8	0	0	2	0	0	30	1	0	0	0
e.	0	0	0	0	0	0	0	0	0	0	0
f.	0	0	0	0	0	0	0	0	0	0	0
10.	0	0	1	0	0	0	1	0	0	0	0
11.	0	0	0	0	0	0	10	3	0	1	1
12.	0	0	0	0	0	0	1	1	0	2	0
13.	0	0	0	0	0	0	0	0	0	0	0
14.	2	0	2	1	0	0	3	3	0	5	1
a.	1	0	1	0	0	0	1	1	0	3	1
b.	0	0	1	0	0	0	0	1	0	2	1
c.	1	0	0	0	0	0	1	1	0	0	0
d.	0	0	0	0	0	0	0	0	0	0	0
15.	72	15	42	29	23	19	209	25	8	26	10
B.	806	97	142	348	155	184	987	292	55	330	111
1.	793	96	141	343	154	182	969	288	54	325	109
2.	8	1	1	3	1	1	10	3	1	3	1
3.	5	0	0	2	0	1	9	1	0	1	1
C.	194	0	20	52	1	16	125	42	0	29	14
1.	47	0	5	13	0	4	30	10	0	11	3
2.	31	0	2	9	0	2	20	7	0	1	2
3.	24	0	3	8	0	3	15	5	0	2	2

Annex Table 2　Mortality by sex, cause and WHO Region, estimates for 1998

DISEASE		WHO MEMBER STATES									
		Both sexes		Males		Females		High income		Low and middle income	
Population (000)		5 884 576		2 963 656		2 920 920		907 828		4 976 748	
		(000)	% total	(000)	% total	(000)	% total	(000)	% total	(000)	% total
4.	Obstructed labour	38	0.1	0	0.0	38	0.1	0	0.0	38	0.1
5.	Abortion	66	0.1	0	0.0	66	0.3	0	0.0	66	0.1
6.	Other maternal conditions	131	0.2	0	0.0	131	0.5	0	0.0	130	0.3
D.	Perinatal conditions	2 155	4.0	1 121	3.9	1 034	4.1	53	0.7	2 102	4.6
E.	Nutritional deficiencies	490	0.9	231	0.8	259	1.0	23	0.3	467	1.0
1.	Protein-energy malnutrition	281	0.5	136	0.5	145	0.6	7	0.1	274	0.6
2.	Iodine deficiency	16	0.0	8	0.0	8	0.0	0	0.0	16	0.0
3.	Vitamin A deficiency	78	0.1	40	0.1	39	0.2	0	0.0	78	0.2
4.	Anaemias	110	0.2	45	0.2	65	0.3	15	0.2	95	0.2
5.	Other nutritional disorders	4	0.0	2	0.0	2	0.0	1	0.0	3	0.0
II.	Noncommunicable conditions	31 717	58.8	16 409	57.6	15 308	60.2	7 024	87.4	24 693	53.8
A.	Malignant neoplasms	7 228	13.4	4 115	14.4	3 113	12.2	2 020	25.1	5 209	11.3
1.	Mouth and oropharynx	352	0.7	233	0.8	120	0.5	41	0.5	312	0.7
2.	Esophagus	436	0.8	289	1.0	147	0.6	49	0.6	387	0.8
3.	Stomach	822	1.5	518	1.8	304	1.2	143	1.8	679	1.5
4.	Colon/rectum	556	1.0	284	1.0	273	1.1	243	3.0	313	0.7
5.	Liver	609	1.1	433	1.5	176	0.7	46	0.6	563	1.2
6.	Pancreas	214	0.4	118	0.4	96	0.4	99	1.2	115	0.3
7.	Trachea/bronchus/lung	1 244	2.3	911	3.2	333	1.3	422	5.3	822	1.8
8.	Melanoma and other skin cancers	55	0.1	28	0.1	27	0.1	25	0.3	30	0.1
9.	Breast	412	0.8	0	0.0	412	1.6	160	2.0	252	0.5
10.	Cervix	237	0.4	0	0.0	237	0.9	17	0.2	220	0.5
11.	Corpus uteri	73	0.1	0	0.0	73	0.3	27	0.3	46	0.1
12.	Ovary	122	0.2	0	0.0	122	0.5	45	0.6	76	0.2
13.	Prostate	239	0.4	239	0.8	0	0.0	115	1.4	124	0.3
14.	Bladder	158	0.3	117	0.4	41	0.2	56	0.7	101	0.2
15.	Lymphoma	248	0.5	144	0.5	104	0.4	91	1.1	157	0.3
16.	Leukaemia	253	0.5	135	0.5	117	0.5	65	0.8	188	0.4
17.	Other cancers	1 199	2.2	666	2.3	532	2.1	373	4.6	825	1.8
B.	Other neoplasms	109	0.2	56	0.2	52	0.2	39	0.5	69	0.2
C.	Diabetes mellitus	600	1.1	257	0.9	343	1.3	161	2.0	439	1.0
D.	Nutritional/endocrine disorders	147	0.3	67	0.2	80	0.3	50	0.6	96	0.2
E.	Neuropsychiatric disorders	720	1.3	380	1.3	340	1.3	225	2.8	495	1.1
1.	Unipolar major disorder	0	0.0	0	0.0	0	0.0	0	0.0	0	0.0
2.	Bipolar affective disorder	16	0.0	5	0.0	11	0.0	1	0.0	15	0.0
3.	Psychoses	54	0.1	29	0.1	25	0.1	14	0.2	40	0.1
4.	Epilepsy	68	0.1	40	0.1	28	0.1	8	0.1	60	0.1
5.	Alcohol dependence	59	0.1	50	0.2	9	0.0	16	0.2	42	0.1
6.	Alzheimer and other dementias	216	0.4	88	0.3	128	0.5	105	1.3	111	0.2
7.	Parkinson disease	63	0.1	34	0.1	29	0.1	33	0.4	30	0.1
8.	Multiple sclerosis	26	0.0	11	0.0	15	0.1	6	0.1	20	0.0
9.	Drug dependence	11	0.0	9	0.0	2	0.0	3	0.0	7	0.0
10.	Post traumatic stress disorder	0	0.0	0	0.0	0	0.0	0	0.0	0	0.0
11.	Obsessive-compulsive disorders	0	0.0	0	0.0	0	0.0	0	0.0	0	0.0
12.	Panic disorder	0	0.0	0	0.0	0	0.0	0	0.0	0	0.0
13.	Other neuropsychiatric disorders	208	0.4	114	0.4	94	0.4	38	0.5	170	0.4

	AFR	AMR High income	AMR Low and middle income	EMR	EUR High income	EUR Low and middle income	SEAR India	SEAR Other low and middle income	WPR High income	WPR China	WPR Other low and middle income
	601 783	*304 886*	*497 925*	*473 644*	*392 402*	*477 727*	*982 223*	*502 833*	*198 497*	*1 255 698*	*196 958*
	(000)	**(000)**	**(000)**	**(000)**	**(000)**	**(000)**	**(000)**	**(000)**	**(000)**	**(000)**	**(000)**
4.	16	0	2	4	0	1	10	3	0	0	1
5.	26	0	5	5	0	2	19	6	0	2	2
6.	51	0	4	14	0	4	31	11	0	11	4
D.	532	11	138	274	20	92	612	203	20	186	66
E.	116	7	60	61	12	22	100	39	4	55	15
1.	79	2	40	39	4	10	53	19	1	25	8
2.	1	0	1	2	0	0	5	1	0	5	1
3.	26	0	4	13	0	3	16	8	0	6	3
4.	10	5	14	6	8	6	26	11	3	18	4
5.	0	0	0	0	0	2	0	0	0	0	0
II.	2 114	2 216	1 933	1 823	3 499	4 266	4 470	2 273	1 285	7 108	729
A.	504	640	427	240	996	778	653	590	379	1 836	184
1.	27	13	15	16	20	26	100	62	8	47	19
2.	27	16	13	11	24	14	62	22	9	231	7
3.	33	45	41	18	71	111	51	44	27	368	13
4.	18	77	28	12	121	76	25	39	45	102	12
5.	65	14	7	12	23	27	16	62	9	355	19
6.	8	31	10	5	49	31	9	9	19	39	3
7.	26	133	48	37	208	184	79	86	80	337	26
8.	9	8	4	2	12	9	1	2	5	1	1
9.	27	51	42	14	79	46	47	29	30	37	9
10.	38	6	30	9	9	19	57	29	3	28	9
11.	4	8	8	2	14	14	4	4	5	8	1
12.	9	14	7	4	22	16	14	10	9	13	3
13.	38	37	25	7	57	18	14	12	21	6	4
14.	16	18	10	10	28	20	8	11	10	23	3
15.	30	29	19	10	45	19	22	22	17	27	7
16.	11	21	15	12	32	23	18	25	12	76	9
17.	118	118	104	58	184	123	124	121	70	139	39
B.	10	13	10	5	19	9	5	7	7	21	2
C.	25	50	96	46	81	49	102	47	29	61	15
D.	23	16	28	14	25	7	2	7	9	13	2
E.	43	72	51	48	111	83	104	53	41	96	17
1.	0	0	0	0	0	0	0	0	0	0	0
2.	1	0	1	1	0	6	2	1	0	2	0
3.	1	5	4	3	7	5	5	4	3	16	1
4.	6	3	6	7	4	8	13	6	1	12	2
5.	5	5	12	1	8	8	5	4	3	5	1
6.	8	33	8	7	53	20	22	14	19	26	5
7.	2	11	2	2	17	8	6	3	6	5	1
8.	1	2	2	1	3	5	3	2	1	6	1
9.	1	1	2	1	2	1	0	1	1	0	0
10.	0	0	0	0	0	0	0	0	0	0	0
11.	0	0	0	0	0	0	0	0	0	0	0
12.	0	0	0	0	0	0	0	0	0	0	0
13.	17	13	14	24	19	22	47	16	7	24	6

Annex Table 2 Mortality by sex, cause and WHO Region, estimates for 1998

DISEASE		WHO MEMBER STATES								
		Both sexes		Males		Females		High income		Low and middle income	
Population (000)		5 884 576		2 963 656		2 920 920		907 828		4 976 748	
		(000)	% total	(000)	% total	(000)	% total	(000)	% total	(000)	% total
F.	Sense organ disorders	20	0.0	11	0.0	9	0.0	0	0.0	20	0.0
1.	Glaucoma	6	0.0	4	0.0	3	0.0	0	0.0	6	0.0
2.	Cataracts	6	0.0	4	0.0	2	0.0	0	0.0	6	0.0
3.	Other sense organ disorders	7	0.0	3	0.0	4	0.0	0	0.0	7	0.0
G.	Cardiovascular diseases	16 690	30.9	8 051	28.2	8 639	34.0	3 592	44.7	13 098	28.5
1.	Rheumatic heart disease	383	0.7	161	0.6	222	0.9	22	0.3	361	0.8
2.	Ischaemic heart disease	7 375	13.7	3 659	12.8	3 717	14.6	1 884	23.5	5 492	12.0
3.	Cerebrovascular disease	5 106	9.5	2 340	8.2	2 766	10.9	893	11.1	4 213	9.2
4.	Inflammatory cardiac disease	548	1.0	276	1.0	272	1.1	74	0.9	474	1.0
5.	Other cardiac diseases	3 277	6.1	1 615	5.7	1 663	6.5	719	9.0	2 558	5.6
H.	Respiratory diseases	2 995	5.6	1 651	5.8	1 344	5.3	391	4.9	2 604	5.7
1.	Chronic obstructive pulmonary disease	2 249	4.2	1 240	4.3	1 010	4.0	280	3.5	1 969	4.3
2.	Asthma	144	0.3	75	0.3	69	0.3	24	0.3	120	0.3
3.	Other respiratory diseases	602	1.1	336	1.2	266	1.0	87	1.1	515	1.1
I.	Digestive diseases	1 783	3.3	1 083	3.8	700	2.8	322	4.0	1 461	3.2
1.	Peptic ulcer disease	174	0.3	104	0.4	70	0.3	33	0.4	141	0.3
2.	Cirrhosis of the liver	775	1.4	534	1.9	241	0.9	122	1.5	653	1.4
3.	Appendicitis	48	0.1	29	0.1	19	0.1	2	0.0	47	0.1
4.	Other digestive diseases	786	1.5	416	1.5	370	1.5	165	2.1	621	1.4
J.	Diseases of the genitourinary system	765	1.4	416	1.5	349	1.4	139	1.7	626	1.4
1.	Nephritis/nephrosis	554	1.0	293	1.0	261	1.0	90	1.1	464	1.0
2.	Benign prostatic hypertrophy	33	0.1	33	0.1	0	0.0	4	0.1	29	0.1
3.	Other genitourinary system diseases	178	0.3	90	0.3	88	0.3	45	0.6	133	0.3
K.	Skin diseases	44	0.1	21	0.1	22	0.1	13	0.2	30	0.1
L.	Musculoskeletal diseases	100	0.2	38	0.1	62	0.2	35	0.4	65	0.1
1.	Rheumatoid arthritis	17	0.0	5	0.0	12	0.0	10	0.1	7	0.0
2.	Osteoarthritis	0	0.0	0	0.0	0	0.0	0	0.0	0	0.0
3.	Other musculoskeletal diseases	83	0.2	33	0.1	50	0.2	25	0.3	58	0.1
M.	Congenital abnormalities	515	1.0	263	0.9	252	1.0	36	0.5	478	1.0
N.	Oral diseases	2	0.0	1	0.0	1	0.0	0	0.0	2	0.0
1.	Dental caries	0	0.0	0	0.0	0	0.0	0	0.0	0	0.0
2.	Periodontal disease	0	0.0	0	0.0	0	0.0	0	0.0	0	0.0
3.	Edentulism	0	0.0	0	0.0	0	0.0	0	0.0	0	0.0
4.	Other oral diseases	2	0.0	1	0.0	1	0.0	0	0.0	2	0.0
III.	Injuries	5 765	10.7	3 815	13.4	1 950	7.7	498	6.2	5 266	11.5
A.	Unintentional	3 493	6.5	2 323	8.1	1 170	4.6	327	4.1	3 166	6.9
1.	Road traffic accidents	1 171	2.2	855	3.0	316	1.2	142	1.8	1 029	2.2
2.	Poisoning	252	0.5	155	0.5	97	0.4	14	0.2	238	0.5
3.	Falls	316	0.6	177	0.6	139	0.5	77	1.0	239	0.5
4.	Fires	282	0.5	119	0.4	163	0.6	11	0.1	271	0.6
5.	Drowning	495	0.9	332	1.2	163	0.6	13	0.2	482	1.1
6.	Other unintentional injuries	977	1.8	685	2.4	293	1.2	70	0.9	907	2.0
B.	Intentional	2 272	4.2	1 491	5.2	780	3.1	172	2.1	2 100	4.6
1.	Self-inflicted	948	1.8	565	2.0	383	1.5	130	1.6	818	1.8
2.	Homicide and violence	736	1.4	582	2.0	153	0.6	38	0.5	698	1.5
3.	War	588	1.1	344	1.2	244	1.0	4	0.0	584	1.3

	AFR	AMR High income	AMR Low and middle income	EMR	EUR High income	EUR Low and middle income	SEAR India	SEAR Other low and middle income	WPR High income	WPR China	WPR Other low and middle income
	601 783	*304 886*	*497 925*	*473 644*	*392 402*	*477 727*	*982 223*	*502 833*	*198 497*	*1 255 698*	*196 958*
	(000)	(000)	(000)	(000)	(000)	(000)	(000)	(000)	(000)	(000)	(000)
F.	0	0	1	0	0	0	0	0	0	18	0
1.	0	0	0	0	0	0	0	0	0	6	0
2.	0	0	0	0	0	0	0	0	0	6	0
3.	0	0	1	0	0	0	0	0	0	6	0
G.	988	1 125	945	1 097	1 802	2 855	2 820	1 102	650	2 951	355
1.	20	7	9	20	11	32	86	8	4	183	3
2.	275	589	420	513	945	1 420	1 471	394	342	881	124
3.	449	281	298	198	449	817	557	325	161	1 467	104
4.	72	23	28	60	37	64	100	59	13	72	20
5.	172	224	190	306	361	522	606	315	129	347	104
H.	220	123	125	133	195	223	284	110	71	1 474	36
1.	110	88	68	64	140	114	153	60	51	1 383	19
2.	14	8	13	8	12	12	21	14	4	34	4
3.	96	27	45	62	43	98	110	37	16	57	12
I.	139	102	142	105	159	152	240	227	59	387	71
1.	12	10	12	5	16	16	41	18	6	32	6
2.	33	39	64	33	59	63	144	99	23	188	30
3.	11	0	2	4	1	2	11	6	0	10	2
4.	83	52	65	62	82	72	44	105	30	158	34
J.	96	44	57	74	70	71	102	77	25	125	25
1.	81	28	42	34	45	30	89	66	16	99	21
2.	1	1	2	1	2	7	11	0	1	7	0
3.	14	14	13	39	23	34	2	10	8	19	3
K.	7	4	4	2	7	2	2	2	2	11	1
L.	1	11	10	2	17	5	3	7	6	36	2
1.	0	3	2	0	5	1	2	1	2	2	0
2.	0	0	0	0	0	0	0	0	0	0	0
3.	1	8	8	2	12	5	1	6	5	34	2
M.	56	14	38	57	16	31	153	45	6	79	19
N.	0	0	0	0	0	0	0	0	0	0	0
1.	0	0	0	0	0	0	0	0	0	0	0
2.	0	0	0	0	0	0	0	0	0	0	0
3.	0	0	0	0	0	0	0	0	0	0	0
4.	0	0	0	0	0	0	0	0	0	0	0
III.	1 163	168	454	463	236	519	923	458	88	1 133	159
A.	566	111	273	198	156	296	723	333	58	661	117
1.	170	49	126	72	66	107	217	119	25	179	41
2.	37	5	5	12	6	48	32	28	2	68	9
3.	20	25	21	10	38	33	50	26	14	70	9
4.	68	4	7	16	5	11	135	7	2	25	3
5.	93	5	29	27	6	29	92	56	2	135	22
6.	179	23	85	61	33	68	199	97	12	185	34
B.	597	58	181	265	81	223	200	125	30	471	41
1.	23	44	28	45	61	102	124	63	24	413	21
2.	266	13	134	55	17	48	72	50	6	58	16
3.	308	0	19	165	2	73	4	12	0	1	4

Annex Table 3 Burden of disease by sex, cause and WHO Region, estimates for 1998

DISEASE		WHO MEMBER STATES								
		Both sexes		Males		Females		High income		Low and middle income	
Population (000)		5 884 576		2 963 656		2 920 920		907 828		4 976 748	
		(000)	% total	(000)	% total	(000)	% total	(000)	% total	(000)	% total
TOTAL DALYs		1 382 564	100	730 815	100	651 749	100	108 305	100	1 274 259	100
I.	Communicable diseases, maternal and perinatal conditions and nutritional deficiencies	565 528	40.9	271 506	37.2	294 022	45.1	7 834	7.2	557 694	43.8
A.	Infectious and parasitic diseases	323 993	23.4	165 383	22.6	158 610	24.3	2 994	2.8	321 000	25.2
1.	Tuberculosis	28 189	2.0	16 137	2.2	12 052	1.8	142	0.1	28 047	2.2
2.	STDs excluding HIV	17 082	1.2	5 855	0.8	11 227	1.7	416	0.4	16 666	1.3
a.	Syphilis	4 967	0.4	2 520	0.3	2 448	0.4	10	0.0	4 957	0.4
b.	Chlamydia	7 150	0.5	1 006	0.1	6 144	0.9	354	0.3	6 796	0.5
c.	Gonorrhoea	4 955	0.4	2 326	0.3	2 629	0.4	46	0.0	4 909	0.4
d.	Other STDs	10	0.0	4	0.0	6	0.0	5	0.0	5	0.0
3.	HIV/AIDS	70 930	5.1	34 985	4.8	35 944	5.5	1 022	0.9	69 907	5.5
4.	Diarrhoeal diseases	73 100	5.3	38 012	5.2	35 089	5.3	359	0.3	72 742	5.7
5.	Childhood diseases	56 855	4.1	29 148	4.0	27 707	4.2	396	0.4	56 459	4.4
a.	Pertussis	13 226	1.0	6 828	0.9	6 398	1.0	179	0.2	13 047	1.0
b.	Polio	213	0.0	117	0.0	96	0.0	0	0.0	213	0.0
c.	Diphtheria	181	0.0	100	0.0	82	0.0	0	0.0	181	0.0
d.	Measles	30 255	2.2	15 526	2.1	14 729	2.3	188	0.2	30 067	2.4
e.	Tetanus	12 979	0.9	6 577	0.9	6 402	1.0	29	0.0	12 950	1.0
6.	Meningitis	4 725	0.3	2 445	0.3	2 280	0.3	154	0.1	4 571	0.4
7.	Hepatitis	1 700	0.1	1 019	0.1	681	0.1	55	0.1	1 645	0.1
8.	Malaria	39 267	2.8	20 188	2.8	19 080	2.9	0	0.0	39 267	3.1
9.	Tropical diseases	10 984	0.8	7 130	1.0	3 854	0.6	6	0.0	10 977	0.9
a.	Trypanosomiasis	1 219	0.1	582	0.1	637	0.1	0	0.0	1 219	0.1
b.	Chagas disease	589	0.0	285	0.0	303	0.0	0	0.0	588	0.0
c.	Schistosomiasis	1 699	0.1	1 004	0.1	695	0.1	3	0.0	1 696	0.1
d.	Leishmaniasis	1 710	0.1	1 057	0.1	653	0.1	3	0.0	1 707	0.1
e.	Lymphatic filariasis	4 698	0.3	3 588	0.5	1 110	0.2	0	0.0	4 698	0.4
f.	Onchocerciasis	1 069	0.1	614	0.1	456	0.1	0	0.0	1 069	0.1
10.	Leprosy	395	0.0	199	0.0	196	0.0	1	0.0	393	0.0
11.	Dengue	558	0.0	257	0.0	302	0.0	0	0.0	558	0.0
12.	Japanese encephalitis	503	0.0	264	0.0	238	0.0	0	0.0	502	0.0
13.	Trachoma	1 263	0.1	342	0.0	921	0.1	8	0.0	1 255	0.1
14.	Intestinal nematode infections	4 279	0.3	2 185	0.3	2 094	0.3	4	0.0	4 275	0.3
a.	Ascariasis	1 292	0.1	662	0.1	630	0.1	1	0.0	1 290	0.1
b.	Trichuriasis	1 287	0.1	660	0.1	628	0.1	0	0.0	1 287	0.1
c.	Hookworm disease	1 698	0.1	863	0.1	835	0.1	2	0.0	1 695	0.1
d.	Other intestinal infections	2	0.0	0	0.0	2	0.0	0	0.0	2	0.0
15.	Other infectious diseases	14 163	1.0	7 218	1.0	6 946	1.1	430	0.4	13 734	1.1
B.	Respiratory infections	85 085	6.2	43 801	6.0	41 284	6.3	1 488	1.4	83 597	6.6
1.	Acute lower respiratory infections	82 344	6.0	42 406	5.8	39 939	6.1	1 355	1.3	80 990	6.4
2.	Acute upper respiratory infections	975	0.1	503	0.1	472	0.1	50	0.0	924	0.1
3.	Otitis media	1 766	0.1	893	0.1	873	0.1	84	0.1	1 683	0.1
C.	Maternal conditions	32 250	2.3	0	0.0	32 250	4.9	398	0.4	31 852	2.5
1.	Haemorrhage	3 833	0.3	0	0.0	3 833	0.6	25	0.0	3 807	0.3
2.	Sepsis	5 965	0.4	0	0.0	5 965	0.9	49	0.0	5 916	0.5
3.	Hypertensive disorders of pregnancy	1 882	0.1	0	0.0	1 882	0.3	18	0.0	1 865	0.1

	AFR	AMR		EMR	EUR		SEAR		WPR		
		High income	Low and middle income		High income	Low and middle income	India	Other low and middle income	High income	China	Other low and middle income
	601 783	*304 886*	*497 925*	*473 644*	*392 402*	*477 727*	*982 223*	*502 833*	*198 497*	*1 255 698*	*196 958*
	(000)	**(000)**	**(000)**	**(000)**	**(000)**	**(000)**	**(000)**	**(000)**	**(000)**	**(000)**	**(000)**
	325 198	35 953	93 907	122 982	51 201	91 496	268 953	121 712	19 998	208 704	42 462
I.	220 309	2 050	25 971	57 276	3 317	15 506	135 263	48 437	2 109	37 779	17 512
A.	159 032	742	13 043	28 450	1 202	5 785	67 619	25 870	900	12 061	9 290
1.	5 442	8	1 213	3 189	53	853	7 577	4 438	80	3 878	1 459
2.	5 249	151	1 231	895	191	545	4 909	2 746	68	111	986
a.	1 980	2	263	375	5	64	1 449	586	1	5	237
b.	1 548	131	663	320	162	372	1 982	1 373	59	73	467
c.	1 721	17	305	199	21	103	1 479	787	7	32	283
d.	0	2	0	0	2	5	0	0	1	0	0
3.	54 101	265	2 348	3 423	402	160	5 611	3 034	353	246	986
4.	24 231	83	3 774	9 510	171	2 056	22 005	6 149	36	2 491	2 594
5.	25 375	11	1 144	6 927	79	1 179	14 463	4 784	256	1 131	1 505
a.	4 793	10	657	1 890	35	581	2 692	1 397	113	606	453
b.	102	0	0	29	0	10	63	0	0	0	10
c.	25	0	3	8	0	24	75	37	0	0	8
d.	17 132	0	17	3 288	30	204	6 474	2 229	143	159	580
e.	3 322	1	467	1 712	15	361	5 160	1 121	0	366	453
6.	791	59	384	452	67	260	1 191	436	23	894	168
7.	253	18	91	167	26	76	300	211	9	475	74
8.	34 506	0	130	1 854	0	0	577	1 608	0	3	588
9.	5 558	1	711	555	3	53	3 204	479	0	255	163
a.	1 141	0	0	77	0	0	0	0	0	0	0
b.	0	0	588	0	0	0	0	0	0	0	0
c.	1 369	0	73	191	1	32	0	8	0	22	3
d.	361	0	37	93	1	18	1 141	42	0	1	15
e.	1 691	0	9	126	0	4	2 063	429	0	232	146
f.	997	0	3	69	0	0	0	0	0	0	0
10.	41	0	51	12	1	3	208	55	0	5	20
11.	16	0	1	1	0	0	353	118	0	21	48
12.	0	0	0	0	0	0	66	83	0	319	34
13.	414	0	0	239	5	90	32	43	0	425	14
14.	495	0	514	168	2	42	797	850	0	1 086	323
a.	78	0	162	58	1	14	163	233	0	489	94
b.	74	0	206	6	0	0	102	308	0	467	124
c.	344	0	147	104	1	27	532	308	0	130	104
d.	0	0	0	0	0	2	0	0	0	0	0
15.	2 559	145	1 451	1 057	202	466	6 325	835	74	720	330
B.	23 369	440	3 525	10 251	726	3 084	25 556	7 161	245	7 790	2 941
1.	22 818	388	3 355	9 953	667	2 960	24 806	6 923	224	7 407	2 844
2.	244	18	45	109	23	43	274	84	8	94	33
3.	307	34	125	189	36	81	475	154	12	289	63
C.	10 251	121	1 694	3 664	188	1 575	7 891	3 201	54	2 536	1 075
1.	1 466	7	160	398	12	116	902	308	3	357	103
2.	1 952	13	292	761	24	327	1 338	563	6	502	189
3.	729	5	99	242	9	76	441	150	2	80	50

Annex Table 3 Burden of disease by sex, cause and WHO Region, estimates for 1998

DISEASE		WHO MEMBER STATES								
		Both sexes		Males		Females		High income		Low and middle income	
Population (000)		5 884 576		2 963 656		2 920 920		907 828		4 976 748	
		(000)	% total	(000)	% total	(000)	% total	(000)	% total	(000)	% total
4.	Obstructed labour	7 040	0.5	0	0.0	7 040	1.1	250	0.2	6 790	0.5
5.	Abortion	5 498	0.4	0	0.0	5 498	0.8	18	0.0	5 479	0.4
6.	Other maternal conditions	8 032	0.6	0	0.0	8 032	1.2	37	0.0	7 995	0.6
D.	Perinatal conditions	80 564	5.8	41 826	5.7	38 737	5.9	2 020	1.9	78 544	6.2
E.	Nutritional deficiencies	43 636	3.2	20 496	2.8	23 140	3.6	935	0.9	42 701	3.4
1.	Protein-energy malnutrition	14 931	1.1	7 441	1.0	7 490	1.1	122	0.1	14 810	1.2
2.	Iodine deficiency	1 078	0.1	544	0.1	534	0.1	23	0.0	1 055	0.1
3.	Vitamin A deficiency	2 801	0.2	1 414	0.2	1 387	0.2	8	0.0	2 793	0.2
4.	Anaemias	24 746	1.8	11 066	1.5	13 680	2.1	773	0.7	23 973	1.9
5.	Other nutritional disorders	80	0.0	32	0.0	49	0.0	9	0.0	71	0.0
II.	Noncommunicable conditions	595 363	43.1	312 942	42.8	282 421	43.3	87 732	81.0	507 631	39.8
A.	Malignant neoplasms	80 837	5.8	45 640	6.2	35 197	5.4	16 257	15.0	64 580	5.1
1.	Mouth and oropharynx	4 473	0.3	2 972	0.4	1 501	0.2	446	0.4	4 027	0.3
2.	Esophagus	4 180	0.3	2 837	0.4	1 343	0.2	398	0.4	3 782	0.3
3.	Stomach	8 156	0.6	5 245	0.7	2 911	0.4	1 049	1.0	7 107	0.6
4.	Colon/rectum	5 191	0.4	2 790	0.4	2 401	0.4	1 818	1.7	3 373	0.3
5.	Liver	7 878	0.6	5 951	0.8	1 926	0.3	391	0.4	7 486	0.6
6.	Pancreas	1 761	0.1	1 062	0.1	699	0.1	669	0.6	1 092	0.1
7.	Trachea/bronchus/lung	11 176	0.8	8 302	1.1	2 874	0.4	3 122	2.9	8 054	0.6
8.	Melanoma and other skin cancers	611	0.0	332	0.0	279	0.0	264	0.2	347	0.0
9.	Breast	5 202	0.4	0	0.0	5 202	0.8	1 643	1.5	3 560	0.3
10.	Cervix	3 183	0.2	0	0.0	3 183	0.5	199	0.2	2 985	0.2
11.	Corpus uteri	705	0.1	0	0.0	705	0.1	199	0.2	506	0.0
12.	Ovary	1 545	0.1	0	0.0	1 545	0.2	403	0.4	1 142	0.1
13.	Prostate	1 551	0.1	1 551	0.2	0	0.0	673	0.6	878	0.1
14.	Bladder	1 392	0.1	1 083	0.1	310	0.0	429	0.4	963	0.1
15.	Lymphoma	3 419	0.2	2 153	0.3	1 266	0.2	759	0.7	2 659	0.2
16.	Leukaemia	4 828	0.3	2 638	0.4	2 190	0.3	630	0.6	4 198	0.3
17.	Other cancers	15 586	1.1	8 725	1.2	6 861	1.1	3 164	2.9	12 421	1.0
B.	Other neoplasms	4 032	0.3	1 957	0.3	2 074	0.3	880	0.8	3 152	0.2
C.	Diabetes mellitus	11 668	0.8	5 489	0.8	6 180	0.9	3 131	2.9	8 537	0.7
D.	Nutritional/endocrine disorders	5 804	0.4	2 664	0.4	3 140	0.5	1 217	1.1	4 588	0.4
E.	Neuropsychiatric disorders	159 462	11.5	78 850	10.8	80 612	12.4	25 414	23.5	134 048	10.5
1.	Unipolar major depression	58 246	4.2	20 674	2.8	37 572	5.8	7 029	6.5	51 217	4.0
2.	Bipolar affective disorder	16 189	1.2	8 237	1.1	7 952	1.2	1 768	1.6	14 421	1.1
3.	Psychoses	14 265	1.0	7 520	1.0	6 745	1.0	2 280	2.1	11 984	0.9
4.	Epilepsy	5 147	0.4	2 812	0.4	2 335	0.4	488	0.5	4 659	0.4
5.	Alcohol dependence	18 292	1.3	16 162	2.2	2 130	0.3	4 739	4.4	13 553	1.1
6.	Alzheimer and other dementias	8 510	0.6	3 671	0.5	4 839	0.7	2 983	2.8	5 527	0.4
7.	Parkinson disease	1 109	0.1	543	0.1	566	0.1	489	0.5	621	0.0
8.	Multiple sclerosis	1 530	0.1	676	0.1	853	0.1	221	0.2	1 308	0.1
9.	Drug dependence	6 326	0.5	5 104	0.7	1 222	0.2	1 544	1.4	4 782	0.4
10.	Post traumatic stress disorder	2 174	0.2	829	0.1	1 346	0.2	278	0.3	1 896	0.1
11.	Obsessive-compulsive disorders	11 566	0.8	5 015	0.7	6 551	1.0	1 504	1.4	10 062	0.8
12.	Panic disorder	5 429	0.4	1 824	0.2	3 605	0.6	719	0.7	4 710	0.4
13.	Other neuropsychiatric disorders	10 678	0.8	5 783	0.8	4 895	0.8	1 370	1.3	9 308	0.7

	AFR	AMR		EMR	EUR		SEAR		WPR		
		High income	Low and middle income		High income	Low and middle income	India	Other low and middle income	High income	China	Other low and middle income
	601 783	*304 886*	*497 925*	*473 644*	*392 402*	*477 727*	*982 223*	*502 833*	*198 497*	*1 255 698*	*196 958*
	(000)	(000)	(000)	(000)	(000)	(000)	(000)	(000)	(000)	(000)	(000)
4.	1 818	86	412	942	116	441	1 601	721	39	621	242
5.	1 788	4	443	412	9	246	1 704	614	2	69	206
6.	2 497	7	289	909	19	368	1 905	845	3	907	284
D.	20 033	434	5 063	10 061	768	3 380	23 316	7 445	762	6 882	2 420
E.	7 624	313	2 648	4 851	432	1 683	10 881	4 760	147	8 511	1 786
1.	4 106	35	1 184	2 200	56	532	3 734	1 298	14	1 218	555
2.	104	9	65	145	10	48	280	77	3	303	33
3.	915	0	128	464	4	99	565	286	0	220	119
4.	2 500	266	1 257	2 042	358	947	6 302	3 098	128	6 770	1 078
5.	0	3	14	0	4	57	0	0	2	0	0
II.	56 353	29 368	50 373	46 549	42 032	60 019	88 657	54 058	15 738	134 185	18 030
A.	7 080	5 269	5 202	3 606	7 825	8 167	8 754	7 600	3 114	21 766	2 454
1.	328	146	194	222	212	325	1 313	696	86	732	220
2.	320	127	117	129	191	152	681	223	78	2 095	67
3.	395	337	388	230	506	1 067	615	489	202	3 778	149
4.	193	580	283	147	883	695	307	401	352	1 224	126
5.	1 023	126	67	170	188	236	176	772	76	4 806	237
6.	98	214	87	56	325	281	102	93	130	347	28
7.	310	996	468	425	1 510	1 766	921	861	607	3 053	258
8.	100	89	52	24	125	102	18	27	50	16	8
9.	336	545	577	232	783	577	711	438	312	552	140
10.	459	67	445	139	94	223	836	413	36	340	131
11.	41	64	93	25	96	133	42	43	38	115	14
12.	127	132	105	69	193	197	206	170	77	212	57
13.	282	208	167	55	332	126	87	92	132	42	27
14.	175	133	91	117	211	186	77	95	83	195	29
15.	648	251	313	215	363	286	360	333	143	392	115
16.	231	217	330	299	296	356	429	594	114	1 740	223
17.	2 015	1 036	1 425	1 053	1 516	1 458	1 874	1 860	599	2 125	625
B.	491	304	475	261	411	434	238	325	161	815	116
C.	486	1 018	1 862	887	1 607	951	1 981	904	494	1 194	285
D.	1 055	433	1 323	779	561	415	96	295	214	522	110
E.	14 144	9 054	17 578	12 053	11 787	14 350	22 944	16 207	4 425	31 517	5 401
1.	5 518	2 511	4 896	4 418	3 243	4 579	9 679	5 912	1 221	14 324	1 946
2.	1 590	639	1 362	1 272	813	1 238	2 746	1 667	299	4 009	552
3.	615	837	1 465	1 299	1 047	1 290	1 964	1 977	380	2 733	658
4.	538	178	642	417	222	456	936	587	83	882	207
5.	2 040	1 736	4 348	373	2 177	1 835	1 074	1 676	822	1 659	551
6.	317	940	715	236	1 469	1 060	922	612	571	1 471	196
7.	49	154	38	49	239	144	138	78	95	102	23
8.	132	79	134	112	102	145	234	143	38	364	47
9.	490	571	1 272	863	704	805	89	804	256	203	269
10.	229	104	190	181	126	168	369	216	47	469	76
11.	1 130	550	976	914	689	927	1 947	1 168	254	2 613	397
12.	528	261	450	410	329	439	882	557	124	1 263	187
13.	968	493	1 091	1 509	627	1 264	1 964	811	233	1 425	292

Annex Table 3 Burden of disease by sex, cause and WHO Region, estimates for 1998

DISEASE	WHO MEMBER STATES									
	Both sexes		Males		Females		High income		Low and middle income	
Population (000)	5 884 576		2 963 656		2 920 920		907 828		4 976 748	
	(000)	% total	(000)	% total	(000)	% total	(000)	% total	(000)	% total
F. Sense organ disorders	12 542	0.9	5 611	0.8	6 931	1.1	158	0.1	12 385	1.0
1. Glaucoma	3 070	0.2	1 188	0.2	1 881	0.3	85	0.1	2 985	0.2
2. Cataracts	9 182	0.7	4 306	0.6	4 876	0.7	68	0.1	9 114	0.7
3. Other sense organ disorders	290	0.0	117	0.0	174	0.0	5	0.0	286	0.0
G. Cardiovascular diseases	143 015	10.3	78 056	10.7	64 959	1.0	19 518	18.0	123 497	9.7
1. Rheumatic heart disease	6 576	0.5	2 929	0.4	3 647	0.6	180	0.2	6 396	0.5
2. Ischaemic heart disease	51 948	3.8	30 044	4.1	21 903	3.4	9 501	8.8	42 447	3.3
3. Cerebrovascular disease	41 626	3.0	21 566	3.0	20 060	3.1	5 219	4.8	36 407	2.9
4. Inflammatory cardiac disease	10 509	0.8	5 675	0.8	4 834	0.7	722	0.7	9 787	0.8
5. Other cardiac diseases	32 356	2.3	17 842	2.4	14 514	2.2	3 896	3.6	28 460	2.2
H. Respiratory diseases	61 603	4.5	33 583	4.6	28 019	4.3	8 050	7.4	53 553	4.2
1. Chronic obstructive pulmonary disease	28 654	2.1	16 393	2.2	12 260	1.9	2 449	2.3	26 205	2.1
2. Asthma	10 968	0.8	6 088	0.8	4 879	0.7	1 208	1.1	9 760	0.8
3. Other respiratory diseases	18 392	1.3	9 651	1.3	8 741	1.3	1 303	1.2	17 089	1.3
I. Digestive diseases	41 111	3.0	24 775	3.4	16 336	2.5	4 365	4.0	36 746	2.9
1. Peptic ulcer disease	2 637	0.2	1 742	0.2	895	0.1	241	0.2	2 395	0.2
2. Cirrhosis of the liver	12 813	0.9	9 184	1.3	3 629	0.6	1 638	1.5	11 175	0.9
3. Appendicitis	1 446	0.1	870	0.1	576	0.1	35	0.0	1 411	0.1
4. Other digestive diseases	24 216	1.8	12 979	1.8	11 237	1.7	2 451	2.3	21 765	1.7
J. Diseases of the genitourinary system	15 576	1.1	9 084	1.2	6 493	1.0	1 220	1.1	14 356	1.1
1. Nephritis/nephrosis	8 429	0.6	4 464	0.6	3 965	0.6	470	0.4	7 959	0.6
2. Benign prostatic hypertrophy	2 150	0.2	2 150	0.3	0	0.0	239	0.2	1 911	0.1
3. Other genitourinary system diseases	4 997	0.4	2 470	0.3	2 528	0.4	511	0.5	4 486	0.4
K. Skin diseases	1 619	0.1	827	0.1	792	0.1	136	0.1	1 482	0.1
L. Musculoskeletal diseases	21 464	1.6	7 939	1.1	13 525	2.1	4 512	4.2	16 952	1.3
1. Rheumatoid arthritis	3 682	0.3	1 021	0.1	2 662	0.4	991	0.9	2 692	0.2
2. Osteoarthritis	15 513	1.1	6 210	0.8	9 303	1.4	3 046	2.8	12 468	1.0
3. Other musculoskeletal diseases	2 269	0.2	708	0.1	1 560	0.2	476	0.4	1 793	0.1
M. Congenital abnormalities	28 147	2.0	14 302	2.0	13 844	2.1	1 915	1.8	26 232	2.1
N. Oral diseases	8 483	0.6	4 165	0.6	4 318	0.7	959	0.9	7 524	0.6
1. Dental caries	4 720	0.3	2 383	0.3	2 337	0.4	432	0.4	4 288	0.3
2. Periodontal disease	295	0.0	148	0.0	147	0.0	36	0.0	258	0.0
3. Edentulism	3 351	0.2	1 603	0.2	1 748	0.3	485	0.4	2 866	0.2
4. Other oral diseases	118	0.0	32	0.0	86	0.0	7	0.0	111	0.0
III. Injuries	221 673	16	146 366	20.0	75 307	11.6	12 739	11.8	208 934	16.4
A. Unintentional	156 184	11.3	103 928	14.2	52 257	8.0	8 972	8.3	147 213	11.6
1. Road traffic accidents	38 849	2.8	28 413	3.9	10 436	1.6	4 556	4.2	34 293	2.7
2. Poisoning	6 364	0.5	3 796	0.5	2 568	0.4	280	0.3	6 085	0.5
3. Falls	27 021	2.0	17 074	2.3	9 947	1.5	1 397	1.3	25 624	2.0
4. Fires	11 967	0.9	4 832	0.7	7 135	1.1	261	0.2	11 706	0.9
5. Drowning	14 896	1.1	10 039	1.4	4 857	0.7	280	0.3	14 616	1.1
6. Other unintentional injuries	57 088	4.1	39 774	5.4	17 314	2.7	2 198	2.0	54 890	4.3
B. Intentional	65 489	4.7	42 438	5.8	23 050	3.5	3 768	3.5	61 721	4.8
1. Self-inflicted	21 511	1.6	12 219	1.7	9 292	1.4	2 416	2.2	19 095	1.5
2. Homicide and violence	21 573	1.6	17 151	2.3	4 421	0.7	1 210	1.1	20 363	1.6
3. War	22 405	1.6	13 068	1.8	9 337	1.4	142	0.1	22 264	1.7

	AFR	AMR		EMR	EUR		SEAR		WPR		
		High income	Low and middle income		High income	Low and middle income	India	Other low and middle income	High income	China	Other low and middle income
	601 783	*304 886*	*497 925*	*473 644*	*392 402*	*477 727*	*982 223*	*502 833*	*198 497*	*1 255 698*	*196 958*
	(000)	(000)	(000)	(000)	(000)	(000)	(000)	(000)	(000)	(000)	(000)
F.	2 240	40	707	942	80	409	3 701	1 548	24	2 379	472
1.	441	26	102	119	41	68	698	481	16	930	145
2.	1 792	12	555	815	37	338	3 001	1 056	7	1 247	322
3.	7	2	50	8	2	3	2	10	1	202	4
G.	12 744	6 109	8 763	13 617	9 553	19 807	26 932	12 728	3 670	24 824	4 269
1.	652	54	189	616	87	563	1 793	106	31	2 450	35
2.	2 867	2 955	3 394	4 500	4 664	9 221	11 697	3 172	1 809	6 690	979
3.	4 894	1 651	2 830	2 244	2 554	5 411	4 814	3 272	986	11 906	1 062
4.	1 536	235	538	1 473	342	896	2 071	1 459	127	1 304	527
5.	2 794	1 214	1 812	4 783	1 906	3 716	6 556	4 719	717	2 473	1 666
H.	4 534	2 634	2 579	2 745	4 111	4 581	5 833	2 272	1 272	30 306	735
1.	1 892	767	1 070	1 110	1 198	1 467	2 536	860	470	17 009	275
2.	1 508	441	1 027	832	551	701	1 525	956	207	2 878	342
3.	4 141	423	1 723	2 869	620	2 158	3 352	1 132	230	1 324	420
I.	4 723	1 435	3 547	3 900	2 072	3 544	5 618	5 417	809	8 276	1 770
1.	294	79	158	123	115	220	853	242	45	429	77
2.	636	545	1 196	598	772	885	2 628	1 704	311	3 006	530
3.	362	12	48	119	16	44	313	176	6	287	63
4.	3 431	799	2 144	3 059	1 168	2 396	1 823	3 296	447	4 553	1 100
J.	2 588	374	1 237	2 457	590	1 716	2 036	1 351	219	2 564	445
1.	1 796	149	608	714	228	445	1 578	903	86	1 616	307
2.	204	74	211	177	114	174	366	185	46	547	52
3.	588	151	418	1 566	249	1 096	92	263	87	401	86
K.	581	44	138	105	66	118	114	71	25	330	26
L.	1 230	1 531	3 579	843	2 116	3 090	1 710	1 829	854	4 113	570
1.	106	338	660	155	467	558	197	173	183	791	55
2.	1 096	1 030	2 538	597	1 424	2 255	1 482	1 447	583	2 617	444
3.	28	163	380	92	224	278	31	209	87	705	72
M.	3 933	791	2 280	3 134	810	1 555	7 454	2 390	289	4 500	1 012
N.	521	332	1 103	1 222	445	882	1 247	1 122	165	1 079	364
1.	357	159	977	612	195	412	783	446	70	558	151
2.	32	13	22	20	17	23	86	30	6	36	10
3.	117	157	95	580	231	443	356	635	87	450	199
4.	16	2	8	11	3	4	22	12	1	35	4
III.	48 536	4 535	17 562	19 156	5 852	15 971	45 032	19 217	2 151	36 740	6 921
A.	28 272	3 233	12 146	9 943	4 112	9 775	39 716	15 635	1 525	26 113	5 713
1.	6 117	1 670	4 411	2 564	2 082	3 213	7 204	3 998	773	5 385	1 433
2.	1 185	100	145	351	129	934	988	735	47	1 491	260
3.	2 205	490	1 700	1 423	648	1 377	10 898	2 808	245	4 175	1 052
4.	3 500	96	304	761	117	321	5 723	334	42	640	129
5.	3 091	101	851	869	126	739	2 703	1 763	45	3 919	689
6.	12 175	776	4 735	3 975	1 010	3 192	12 201	5 997	373	10 503	2 151
B.	20 264	1 302	5 416	9 213	1 739	6 195	5 316	3 582	626	10 627	1 208
1.	646	858	708	1 266	1 117	2 071	3 337	1 686	424	8 837	560
2.	7 878	443	3 986	1 649	552	1 319	1 847	1 445	202	1 764	488
3.	11 740	1	722	6 298	71	2 805	132	451	0	26	160

Annex Table 4 Leading causes of mortality and burden of disease, estimates for 1998

	Mortality in all Member States				DALYs in all Member States		
	Rank	% of total	(000)		Rank	% of total	(000)
Both sexes				**Both sexes**			
Ischaemic heart disease	1	13.7	7 375	Acute lower respiratory infections	1	6.0	82 344
Cerebrovascular disease	2	9.5	5 106	Perinatal conditions	2	5.8	80 564
Acute lower respiratory infections	3	6.4	3 452	Diarrhoeal diseases	3	5.3	73 100
HIV/AIDS	4	4.2	2 285	HIV/AIDS	4	5.1	70 930
Chronic obstructive pulmonary disease	5	4.2	2 249	Unipolar major depression	5	4.2	58 246
Diarrhoeal diseases	6	4.1	2 219	Ischaemic heart disease	6	3.8	51 948
Perinatal conditions	7	4.0	2 155	Cerebrovascular disease	7	3.0	41 626
Tuberculosis	8	2.8	1 498	Malaria	8	2.8	39 267
Cancer of trachea/bronchus/lung	9	2.3	1 244	Road traffic accidents	9	2.8	38 849
Road traffic accidents	10	2.2	1 171	Measles	10	2.2	30 255
Males				**Males**			
Ischaemic heart disease	1	12.8	3 659	Acute lower respiratory infections	1	5.8	42 406
Cerebrovascular disease	2	8.2	2 340	Perinatal conditions	2	5.7	41 826
Acute lower respiratory infections	3	6.1	1 753	Diarrhoeal diseases	3	5.2	38 012
Chronic obstructive pulmonary disease	4	4.3	1 240	HIV/AIDS	4	4.8	34 985
HIV/AIDS	5	4.1	1 164	Ischaemic heart disease	5	4.1	30 044
Diarrhoeal diseases	6	4.0	1 149	Road traffic accidents	6	3.9	28 413
Perinatal conditions	7	3.9	1 121	Cerebrovascular disease	7	3.0	21 566
Cancer of trachea/bronchus/lung	8	3.2	911	Unipolar major depression	8	2.8	20 674
Tuberculosis	9	3.1	893	Malaria	9	2.8	20 188
Road traffic accidents	10	3.0	855	Homicide and violence	10	2.3	17 151
Females				**Females**			
Ischaemic heart disease	1	14.6	3 717	Acute lower respiratory infections	1	6.1	39 939
Cerebrovascular disease	2	10.9	2 766	Perinatal conditions	2	5.9	38 737
Acute lower respiratory infections	3	6.7	1 699	Unipolar major depression	3	5.8	37 572
HIV/AIDS	4	4.4	1 121	HIV/AIDS	4	5.5	35 944
Diarrhoeal diseases	5	4.2	1 070	Diarrhoeal diseases	5	5.4	35 089
Perinatal conditions	6	4.1	1 034	Ischaemic heart disease	6	3.4	21 903
Chronic obstructive pulmonary disease	7	4.0	1 010	Cerebrovascular disease	7	3.1	20 060
Tuberculosis	8	2.4	605	Malaria	8	2.9	19 080
Malaria	9	2.1	538	Measles	9	2.3	14 729
Measles	10	1.7	432	Congenital abnormalities	10	2.1	13 844

Leading causes of mortality and DALYs in all Member States and their ranks in WHO Regions

	All Member States		Africa		The Americas		Eastern Mediterranean		Europe		South-East Asia		Western Pacific	
	rank	% of total	rank	% of total	rank	% of total	rank	% of total	rank	% of total	rank	% of total	rank	% of total
Deaths														
Ischaemic heart disease	1	13.7	9	2.9	1	17.9	1	13.6	1	25.5	1	13.8	3	11.1
Cerebrovascular disease	2	9.5	7	4.7	2	10.3	5	5.3	2	13.7	4	6.5	1	14.3
Acute lower respiratory infections	3	6.4	3	8.2	3	4.2	2	9.1	4	3.6	2	9.3	4	4.0
HIV/AIDS	4	4.2	1	19.0	13	1.8	27	0.4	42	0.2	8	2.2	42	0.2
Chronic obstructive pulmonary disease	5	4.2	14	1.1	6	2.8	10	1.7	5	2.7	11	1.6	2	12.0
Diarrhoeal diseases	6	4.1	4	7.6	10	2.0	3	7.4	22	0.7	3	6.6	17	1.2
Perinatal conditions	7	4.0	5	5.5	7	2.6	4	7.3	13	1.2	5	6.0	10	2.2
Tuberculosis	8	2.8	11	2.2	19	1.0	7	3.7	23	0.6	6	5.1	9	2.9
Trachea/bronchus/lung	9	2.3	38	0.3	4	3.2	20	1.0	3	4.2	15	1.2	6	3.6
Road traffic accidents	10	2.2	12	1.8	5	3.1	9	1.9	8	1.9	7	2.5	12	2.0
DALYs														
Acute lower respiratory infections	1	6.0	4	7.0	9	2.9	2	8.1	8	2.5	1	8.1	4	3.9
Perinatal conditions	2	5.8	5	6.2	5	4.2	1	8.2	5	2.9	2	7.9	5	3.7
Diarrhoeal diseases	3	5.3	3	7.5	8	3.0	3	7.7	17	1.6	3	7.2	13	1.9
HIV/AIDS	4	5.1	1	16.6	13	2.0	7	2.8	46	0.4	12	2.2	36	0.6
Unipolar major depression	5	4.2	11	1.7	1	5.7	6	3.6	3	5.5	4	4.0	2	6.5
Ischaemic heart disease	6	3.8	20	0.9	2	4.9	5	3.7	1	9.7	5	3.8	7	3.5
Cerebrovascular disease	7	3.0	13	1.5	6	3.5	12	1.8	2	5.6	13	2.1	3	5.1
Malaria	8	2.8	2	10.6	80	0.1	16	1.5	97	0.0	39	0.6	60	0.2
Road traffic accidents	9	2.8	9	1.9	4	4.7	11	2.1	4	3.7	8	2.9	9	2.8
Measles	10	2.2	6	5.3	92	0.0	8	2.7	67	0.2	11	2.2	48	0.3

Annex Table 5 Demographic characteristics of WHO Regions, estimates for 1978 and 1998

Demographic characteristics	Year	Total population (000 000)	Dependency ratio (per100)	Number of live births (000)	Total fertility rate	Number of deaths (000)	Death rate (per 1 000)	Probability of dying before age 5 (per 1 000)	Life expectancy at birth (years)	GDP per capita adjusted for purchasing power in 1985 US$[a] (US$)
WHO Member States										
Total	1978	4 281	72	120 129	3.9	46 793	11.0	124	61	...
	1998	5 885	59	129 434	2.7	53 929	9.2	83	66	...
High income	1978	793	54	11 519	1.9	7 099	9.0	19	73	11 855
	1998	901	49	10 668	1.7	8 033	8.8	8	78	15 142
China	1978	972	73	20 246	3.3	6 641	6.7	...	65	823
	1998	1 256	47	20 135	1.8	9 296	7.4	48	70	1 493
India	1978	661	76	22 695	4.8	9 066	13.9	...	53	882
	1998	982	64	24 672	3.1	9 337	9.5	89	63	1 282
Other low and middle income	1978	1 855	79	65 669	4.8	23 988	13.0	149	58	...
	1998	2 745	67	73 959	3.4	27 263	9.9	100	61	...
Africa										
	1978	348	94	16 440	6.7	6 386	18.4	208	47	1 524
	1998	602	90	24 073	5.4	9 621	16.0	161	49	1 261
The Americas										
High income	1978	250	52	3 777	1.8	2 115	8.5	18	73	15 266
	1998	305	52	4 140	1.9	2 538	8.3	8	77	17 788
Low and middle income	1978	341	81	11 286	4.5	2 959	8.8	93	63	4 024
	1998	497	61	11 437	2.7	3 113	6.3	46	69	4 248
Eastern Mediterranean										
	1978	272	90	12 142	6.5	3 877	14.5	185	54	2 081
	1998	474	78	15 265	4.4	3 773	8.0	104	63	2 139
Europe										
High income	1978	368	57	4 788	1.9	3 870	10.5	18	73	10 207
	1998	392	49	4 120	1.5	3 974	10.1	8	78	13 081
Low and middle income	1978	419	55	8 277	2.5	4 241	10.1	51	68	...
	1998	478	51	6 449	1.8	5 281	11.1	39	68	...
South-East Asia										
India	1978	661	76	22 695	4.8	9 066	13.9	...	53	882
	1998	982	64	24 672	3.1	9 337	9.5	89	63	1 282
Other low and middle income	1978	352	85	13 048	5.1	5 051	14.5	163	53	1 249
	1998	503	58	11 753	2.6	4 147	8.2	83	63	2 208
Western Pacific										
High income	1978	172	52	2 864	2.1	1 095	6.4	22	73	9 602
	1998	198	44	2 305	1.5	1 482	7.5	9	78	14 890
China	1978	972	73	20 246	3.3	6 641	6.7	...	65	823
	1998	1 256	47	20 135	1.8	9 296	7.4	48	70	1 493
Other low and middle income	1978	126	85	4 566	5.2	1 493	11.9	127	57	...
	1998	197	69	5 085	3.3	1 367	7.0	58	67	...

...Data not available or not applicable.

[a] Estimates for 1978 and 1992.

Annex Table 6 Country performance on infant mortality and female life expectancy: outcomes relative to income, 1952–1992

Selected countries by WHO Regions	Infant mortality rate Percentage higher (lower) than predicted					Female life expectancy Years higher (lower) than predicted				
	1952	1962	1972	1982	1992	1952	1962	1972	1982	1992
Africa										
Algeria	...	31	32	31	11	...	-1.4	0.2	1.4	5.3
Angola	...	42	45	44	55	...	-13.6	-13.9	-11.1	-9.1
Benin	...	29	21	19	26	...	-9.9	-7.6	-5.4	-4.1
Botswana	...	-21	-28	-14	0	...	2.4	2.7	2.6	0.4
Burkina Faso	...	14	14	21	35	...	-7.6	-6.2	-6.8	-9.5
Burundi	...	7	14	20	52	...	-3.4	-3.1	-4	-12.8
Cameroon	...	11	1	15	22	...	-5.5	-4.7	-4.8	-3.5
Cape Verde	...	-28	-28	-12	-5	...	8.6	8.5	8.2	9.9
Central African Republic	...	19	11	17	32	...	-5.7	-5.9	-5.5	-6.7
Chad	...	33	34	39	52	...	-11.1	-10.6	-9.1	-6.7
Comoros	...	14	7	9	14	...	-0.7	-0.5	0.6	3.2
Congo	...	2	-7	17	52	...	-4.4	-5.4	-5.9	-11.1
Côte d'Ivoire	...	22	25	33	35	...	-7.7	-7.7	-7.4	-9.7
Ethiopia	31	34	29	46	...	-4.4	-4.4	-4.5	-7.2	...
Gabon	...	42	66	87	81	...	-8.6	-10.9	-11.4	-9.9
Gambia	...	40	42	52	62	...	-12.3	-13.3	-14.1	-11.2
Ghana	...	-5	-5	-3	5	...	-1.2	-1.2	-0.7	1.4
Guinea	...	35	38	50	63	...	-12	-12.2	-14.5	-12.6
Guinea-Bissau	...	35	43	52	66	...	-10.2	-13.5	-13.2	-11.6
Kenya	-11	-16	-19	-14	-4	-0.1	0.8	1.6	1.7	0.0
Lesotho	...	7	8	25	35	...	2.8	2.0	-0.8	0.8
Liberia	...	27	47	21	...	...	-3.9	-3.8	-3.7	...
Madagascar	...	30	31	19	24	...	-6.8	-5.5	-3.3	0.2
Malawi	...	40	46	52	70	...	-5.9	-7.8	-8.1	-13
Mali	...	40	53	49	52	...	-6.6	-5	-5.7	-3
Mauritania	...	23	20	23	35	...	-7.4	-7.2	-7.1	-4.7
Mauritius	-4	-37	-39	-61	-53	3.9	9.0	8.8	7.7	8.8
Mozambique	...	38	50	39	48	...	-9.8	-10.5	-10.5	-7.6
Namibia	...	23	38	40	24	...	-6.5	-6.8	-6.5	-3.2
Niger	...	29	35	42	54	...	-9.3	-11.2	-10.8	-7.4
Nigeria	-6	-4	-1	19	22	-3.9	-4.7	-6.8	-10.3	-7.6
Rwanda	...	5	17	26	63	...	-1.6	-4.5	-7.2	-33.5
Senegal	...	26	10	-2	2	...	-9.5	-9.1	-9	-6.9
Sierra Leone	...	48	57	75	102	...	-15.4	-17.1	-20.1	-22.6
Somalia	...	34	29	42	84	...	-11.2	-9.7	-11.4	-17.6
South Africa	-31	-16	3	16	25	-1	-0.1	-0.5	-0.9	0.1
Swaziland	...	27	43	44	38	...	-7.2	-6.6	-6	-2.7
Togo	...	22	7	9	21	...	-2.7	-3.3	-2.9	-5
Trinidad and Tobago	-30	-23	-7	4	-41	11.5	12.8	9.5	9.3	9.6
Uganda	-5	-11	-3	21	48	-1.2	-1.3	-2.9	-7	-17.8
United Republic of Tanzania	...	7	4	1	17	...	-0.7	-0.8	-0.7	-4.8
Zambia	...	-2	-10	-4	17	...	-4.5	-4.5	-4.1	-12.7
Zimbabwe	...	-21	-18	-14	1	...	-1.1	0.0	0.0	-6.6
The Americas										
Argentina	-32	-15	-8	-22	-36	16.3	14.8	12.4	11.1	11.0
Barbados	...	-40	-60	-83	-59	...	15.6	14.1	12.8	12.4
Belize	...	...	...	-35	-23	...	...	...	11.1	11.1
Bolivia	18	26	42	38	23	-3.4	-4.2	-5.9	-3.9	-0.2
Brazil	-10	-2	8	21	19	7.0	6.4	5.8	4.8	5.7
Chile	2	19	1	-83	-98	9.0	8.1	9.3	12.6	13.0
Colombia	-15	-21	-21	-27	-23	6.1	8.5	8.0	9.4	9.4
Costa Rica	-42	-26	-39	-108	-112	12.3	12.7	13.4	14.7	14.4
Dominican Republic	-6	-6	-7	1	-24	2.4	5.2	7.0	7.7	9.4
Ecuador	-8	-1	0	13	4	4.1	5.5	5.1	5.6	8.4
El Salvador	0	3	10	4	-37	0.9	3.4	5.2	4.1	9.5
Guatemala	-1	11	10	16	-6	-4	-3.2	-0.3	0.0	3.4
Guyana	-14	-21	-20	-11	-4	7.2	8.1	6.9	5.0	6.5
Haiti	...	28	27	28	6	...	-3.9	-2.3	-3.8	-2.5
Honduras	6	5	-4	-24	-39	-1.6	0.4	2.3	5.3	9.6

Selected countries by WHO Regions	Infant mortality rate Percentage higher (lower) than predicted					Female life expectancy Years higher (lower) than predicted				
	1952	1962	1972	1982	1992	1952	1962	1972	1982	1992
Jamaica	...	-61	-58	-79	-75	...	16.2	14.1	12.6	13.1
Mexico	-1	-4	7	14	10	5.0	7.8	7.5	8.6	9.5
Nicaragua	14	13	12	6	-29	-1.9	-1.1	0.7	3.1	8.4
Panama	-47	-61	-65	-67	-62	10.5	12.1	11.5	11.9	11.7
Paraguay	-73	-70	-68	-35	-25	19.1	16.4	13.7	9.2	8.8
Peru	12	25	31	27	5	-1.4	-1.2	0.7	2.9	6.8
Suriname	...	-50	-48	-30	-39	...	10.7	9.8	8.1	8.5
Uruguay	-51	-46	-35	-31	-57	20.7	18.1	14.6	12.3	12.3
Venezuela	31	31	17	2	-21	7.3	8.2	10.0	8.8	9.5
Eastern Mediterranean										
Bahrain	...	...	...	-1	-7	...	...	...	7.9	8.3
Djibouti	...	...	47	46	...	...	...	-12.7	-11.7	...
Egypt	19	25	31	36	10	-0.1	0.3	-0.1	-0.9	3.9
Iran, Islamic Republic of	...	57	72	41	-1	...	-2.1	-2.5	1.2	4.3
Iraq	...	44	46	70	...	...	-2.3	0.0	0.5	...
Jordan	...	-1	-16	-5	-32	...	-0.3	3.0	4.4	6.1
Morocco	10	15	14	23	13	-0.3	0.4	0.4	0.7	4.0
Oman	...	...	108	41	16	...	...	-8.3	1.8	6.3
Pakistan	12	11	20	25	28	-5.3	-2.8	-2.3	-0.1	2.2
Saudi Arabia	...	78	99	105	8	...	-6.6	-3.5	0.5	6.0
Sudan	...	...	-6	-1	17	...	...	-7	-5.5	-5.2
Syrian Arab Republic	...	10	3	17	0	...	2.4	2.5	2.5	5.1
Tunisia	...	19	15	5	-31	...	0.4	1.6	3.3	5.5
Yemen	...	...	45	38	48	...	...	-9.7	-8.5	-5.9
Europe										
Bulgaria	...	...	...	-105	-56	...	...	...	12.4	9.6
Greece	-88	-72	-62	-99	-113	21.4	19.2	16.4	14.9	14.6
Hungary	...	...	-71	-81	-94	...	...	15.0	10.7	9.1
Malta	...	-128	-138	-133	-106	...	20.4	16.7	13.8	13.3
Poland	...	...	-101	-90	-83	...	...	17.0	13.0	11.6
Romania	...	-84	-108	-116	-83	...	22.9	19.3	14.2	11.2
Turkey	43	43	45	49	25	-0.4	2.6	4.0	3.8	5.8
Yugoslavia	...	-29	-44	-22	-51	...	14.0	13.4	10.2	9.9
South-East Asia										
Bangladesh	...	13	23	35	36	...	-9.6	-9.3	-7.8	-4.9
India	12	14	11	13	17	-4.9	-3.3	-2.5	-1.3	0.6
Indonesia	...	-4	-4	5	4	...	-4	-0.9	0.1	2.7
Myanmar	30	12	2	9	20	-0.6	2.6	2.7	1.0	3.6
Nepal	...	31	29	30	...	...	-8.7	-8.6	-8.1	...
Sri Lanka	-53	-45	-66	-99	-96	10.3	13.7	12.2	12.2	12.1
Thailand	-21	-34	-46	-49	-32	4.9	7.3	7.1	7.8	8.0
Western Pacific										
China	...	-14	-67	-58	-33	...	4.2	12.9	11.4	10.1
Fiji	...	-45	-61	-58	-58	...	9.8	10.2	9.5	9.7
Lao People's Democratic Republic	...	...	...	...	58	...	...	...	...	-8.3
Malaysia	...	-65	-77	-67	-81	...	6.8	9.0	8.4	8.3
Mongolia	...	...	...	...	3	...	...	...	...	3.3
Papua New Guinea	...	23	6	-8	10	...	-7.9	-7.9	-6.4	-4.2
Philippines	-50	-52	-38	-24	-40	5.0	6.5	5.0	4.4	6.9
Solomon Islands	...	...	...	-76	-71	...	...	...	11.0	10.6
Vanuatu	...	...	...	...	-24	...	...	...	...	6.2

... Data not available or not applicable.

Notes:

1. The performance measures in this table are based on the difference between a country's actual level of the health indicator and what would be predicted given its income level. As health indicators at any given income level have improved markedly over the 40 years covered, the predictions are period specific. The Explanatory Notes of the Annex provide more information on data and methods.

2. A country's performance relative to income depends on many factors – education levels, environmental conditions and health policies, to name a few. The reported measures do not, therefore, assess health policies per se but rather provide a quantitative outcome measure to facilitate discussion of health policy.

3. Entries in the table relate each country's actual levels of infant mortality and female life expectancy to what would be predicted given its income level and at the indicated time. Performance on infant mortality is measured as the percentage higher (or lower) than the actual rate relative to the predicted rate; negative numbers therefore indicate better performance. Performance on female life expectancy is years more (or less) than predicted and negative numbers indicate worse performance.

Annex Table 7 Country performance on equity: health conditions of advantaged and disadvantaged groups, around 1990

Country	Percentage of population in absolute poverty	Probability of dying (per 100) between ages 15 and 59				Probability of dying (per 1000) between birth and age 5				Prevalence of tuberculosis (per 100)	
		Males		Females		Males		Females			
		Non-poor	Poor: non-poor ratio	Non-poor	Poor: non-poor ratio	Non-poor	Poor: non-poor ratio	Non-poor	Poor: non-poor ratio	Non-poor	Poor: non-poor ratio
Aggregate		19	2.2	9	4.3	39	4.3	38	4.8	23	2.6
Africa											
Botswana	33	22	2.3	13	4.0	38	4.9	33	4.8	54	1.2
Côte d'Ivoire	18	44	1.5	41	1.5	124	2.4	95	3.3	30	1.6
Ethiopia	46	30	2.2	19	3.6	107	3.0	76	4.0	19	2.9
Guinea	88	22	2.1	12	3.5	66	3.7	45	5.6	20	1.9
Guinea-Bissau	26	37	1.7	30	2.1	177	2.2	135	3.0	20	2.6
Kenya	50	24	2.1	13	3.8	43	3.7	41	3.8	21	2.6
Lesotho	49	15	2.6	7	5.4	58	3.9	43	5.2	45	1.7
Madagascar	72	20	2.0	11	3.4	46	3.8	39	4.1	17	2.6
Mauritania	31	28	1.9	17	3.4	105	3.0	85	3.7	49	1.3
Niger	62	26	1.9	14	3.5	88	3.4	60	4.8	17	2.4
Nigeria	31	32	1.8	22	2.8	101	3.1	82	3.7	27	2.2
Rwanda	46	79	1.2	83	1.0	133	2.7	90	4.2	18	2.3
Senegal	54	27	2.2	14	3.8	49	4.0	39	4.9	21	2.5
South Africa	24	35	1.7	16	3.6	47	4.7	31	5.3	61	1.0
United Republic of Tanzania	11	24	2.1	16	3.3	36	5.6	34	5.0	30	1.4
Uganda	69	46	1.4	41	1.4	131	2.1	111	2.5	38	1.3
Zambia	85	29	2.5	18	3.6	48	3.5	42	3.9	22	3.8
Zimbabwe	41	35	2.1	30	2.3	51	4.1	38	5.0	58	1.2
The Americas											
Brazil	24	23	2.4	6	7.9	26	6.5	23	5.0	6	5.3
Chile	15	12	3.7	3	12.3	10	7.1	7	8.3	2	8.0
Colombia	7	25	2.1	10	5.2	39	5.6	29	6.8	6	7.7
Costa Rica	19	7	5.5	3	10.6	10	5.5	8	5.1	2	4.8
Dominican Republic	20	12	3.4	5	9.7	29	6.5	24	6.5	10	4.6
Ecuador	8	18	2.7	11	4.4	58	4.2	45	4.9	25	1.8
Guatemala	53	23	1.9	9	3.5	31	3.5	29	3.3	8	1.8
Honduras	47	15	2.0	7	4.0	32	3.2	26	3.2	11	1.8
Jamaica	4	13	3.4	7	7.2	26	7.5	19	10.0	1	25.1
Mexico	15	16	2.9	5	8.6	23	7.6	19	7.8	4	6.7
Nicaragua	44	16	2.1	6	5.6	32	3.8	26	4.0	8	2.1
Panama	26	9	3.7	4	7.7	14	6.2	14	5.8	5	3.9
Peru	49	16	1.7	6	3.6	37	3.6	30	3.7	15	2.9
Venezuela	12	16	3.0	6	7.6	16	8.9	11	10.8	3	8.7
Eastern Mediterranean											
Egypt	8	20	2.5	12	4.1	72	3.2	71	3.5	2	16.9
Pakistan	12	18	2.8	12	4.4	105	2.7	101	2.8	39	1.3
Tunisia	4	25	2.2	14	3.8	79	2.8	61	3.7	10	4.3
Europe											
Czech Republic	3	20	2.3	8	6.4	10	17.3	5	29.3	1	31.0
Estonia	6	30	1.8	8	6.3	22	9.3	9	17.5	6	7.5
Kyrgyzstan	19	23	2.1	6	8.0	30	5.7	22	6.1	9	5.1
Poland	7	23	2.2	7	7.8	10	15.7	8	14.4	4	10.9
Romania	18	20	2.3	5	8.4	16	9.9	12	9.2	12	3.9
Slovakia	13	22	2.3	5	9.8	7	11.1	6	11.0	2	7.8
Turkmenistan	5	40	2.2	36	2.4	65	4.2	61	4.0	24	2.2
South-East Asia											
India	53	16	2.1	8	3.7	33	4.5	40	4.3	28	2.5
Indonesia	12	23	2.3	17	3.1	62	4.1	53	4.1	82	0.7
Nepal	50	21	2.2	13	3.8	52	4.0	53	4.6	21	3.3
Sri Lanka	4	18	2.7	9	5.7	18	10.8	19	8.7	6	6.9
Western Pacific											
China	22	12	3.4	4	11.0	23	5.9	28	6.6	14	3.8
Malaysia	6	18	3.1	10	5.1	13	13.7	10	15.0	13	3.2
Philippines	29	15	2.9	7	6.1	23	5.8	18	5.9	71	0.8

Annex Table 8 Malaria: magnitude of the problem by age, sex and WHO Region, estimates for 1998

	Both sexes	Males					Females				
		0–4	5–14	15–44	45–59	60+	0–4	5–14	15–44	45–59	60+
Deaths (000)											
All Member States	1 110	417	105	40	6	3	376	104	46	7	4
Africa	961	391	85	20	1	1	354	84	25	1	1
The Americas	4	0	0	1	0	0	0	0	1	0	0
Eastern Mediterranean	53	19	5	2	0	0	17	5	3	0	0
Europe	0	0	0	0	0	0	0	0	0	0	0
South-East Asia	73	6	11	14	4	2	4	11	15	4	2
Western Pacific	20	1	4	4	1	1	1	3	3	1	1
Incidence (000)											
All Member States	272 925	51 627	23 457	55 786	3 677	2 025	50 847	23 225	56 049	3 854	2 379
Africa	237 647	47 798	19 624	47 923	2 292	1 221	47 132	19 465	48 290	2 441	1 461
The Americas	2 043	121	236	500	111	70	112	218	483	112	80
Eastern Mediterranean	13 693	2 437	1 242	2 841	222	128	2 398	1 226	2 822	227	149
Europe	0	0	0	0	0	0	0	0	0	0	0
South-East Asia	15 791	1 042	1 871	3 627	850	472	994	1 850	3 677	878	529
Western Pacific	3 751	228	483	895	203	134	211	465	777	196	160
DALYs (000)											
All Member States	39 267	14 826	3 916	1 322	97	26	13 551	3 870	1 510	114	33
Africa	34 506	13 889	3 151	696	18	5	12 723	3 137	857	24	7
The Americas	130	11	19	32	4	1	10	17	31	4	1
Eastern Mediterranean	1 854	676	192	77	7	1	619	190	82	7	2
Europe	0	0	0	0	0	0	0	0	0	0	0
South-East Asia	2 185	198	417	410	55	14	161	405	444	64	17
Western Pacific	591	52	137	107	15	4	38	121	96	16	6

Annex Table 9 Tobacco: magnitude of the problem by sex and WHO Region, estimates for 1998

Deaths (000)	Both sexes	Males	Females	DALYs (000)	Both sexes	Males	Females
All Member States	4 023	3 241	782	**All Member States**	49 288	40 037	9 251
Africa	125	112	13	Africa	1 900	1 763	137
The Americas	582	413	169	The Americas	6 787	4 875	1 912
High income	414	283	131	High income	4 523	3 098	1 425
Low and middle income	168	130	38	Low and middle income	2 264	1 777	487
Eastern Mediterranean	182	160	22	Eastern Mediterranean	2 976	2 547	429
Europe	1 369	1 066	303	Europe	18 141	14 396	3 744
High income	635	425	210	High income	6 944	4 654	2 290
Low and middle income	735	641	94	Low and middle income	11 196	9 742	1 454
South-East Asia	580	505	75	South-East Asia	7 439	6 456	983
India	383	332	51	India	5 098	4 415	683
Other low and middle income	197	173	24	Other low and middle income	2 341	2 041	300
Western Pacific	1 185	986	200	Western Pacific	12 044	9 998	2 046
High income	209	147	62	High income	2 296	1 623	673
China	913	783	130	China	8 991	7 716	1 275
Other low and middle income	64	56	8	Other low and middle income	757	659	98

Annex Table 10 Tuberculosis: magnitude of the problem by sex and WHO Region, estimates for 1998

| | Individuals infected with tuberculosis, who are | | | | | |
| | HIV positive | | | HIV negative | | |
	Both sexes	Males	Females	Both sexes	Males	Females
Deaths (000)						
All Member States	**365**	**184**	**181**	**1 498**	**893**	**605**
Africa	305	147	158	209	101	108
The Americas						
High income	1	1	0	1	1	0
Low and middle income	13	7	6	53	30	23
Eastern Mediterranean	3	2	1	139	88	51
Europe						
High income	3	2	1	7	4	2
Low and middle income	1	1	0	53	44	9
South-East Asia						
India	26	18	9	421	281	140
Other low and middle income	9	5	4	261	133	128
Western Pacific						
High income	0	0	0	10	7	3
China	3	2	1	259	161	97
Other low and middle income	2	1	1	86	44	42
Incidence (000)						
All Member States	**619**	**313**	**306**	**7 393**	**4 420**	**2 973**
Africa	510	246	264	1 047	505	543
The Americas						
High income	4	3	1	17	12	6
Low and middle income	22	12	10	378	213	165
Eastern Mediterranean	4	3	2	607	384	223
Europe						
High income	8	5	3	72	48	24
Low and middle income	2	2	0	357	295	62
South-East Asia						
India	46	31	15	1 794	1 198	596
Other low and middle income	16	8	8	1 146	584	562
Western Pacific						
High income	1	0	0	86	57	29
China	5	3	2	1 411	881	530
Other low and middle income	3	2	2	478	243	234
DALYs (000)						
All Member States	**9 032**	**4 365**	**4 667**	**28 189**	**16 137**	**12 052**
Africa	7 934	3 719	4 215	5 442	2 551	2 891
The Americas						
High income	7	5	2	8	6	2
Low and middle income	302	159	143	1 213	638	575
Eastern Mediterranean	59	37	22	3 188	2 006	1 182
Europe						
High income	20	14	6	53	38	15
Low and middle income	18	15	3	853	732	122
South-East Asia						
India	476	303	174	7 577	4 815	2 761
Other low and middle income	154	78	75	4 438	2 264	2 174
Western Pacific						
High income	2	1	1	80	58	22
China	37	22	15	3 878	2 286	1 592
Other low and middle income	25	13	12	1 459	744	715

INDEX

Page numbers in **bold** type indicate main discussions.